ANGEL WINGS

ANGEL WINGS

Air Evac Nursing

Dori E. Childress, R.N., M.S.N.

VANTAGE PRESS
New York

FIRST EDITION

Published by Vantage Press, Inc.
516 West 34th Street, New York, New York 10001

Manufactured in the United States of America
ISBN: 0-533-12259-7

Library of Congress Catalog Card No.: 96-91042

0 9 8 7 6 5 4 3 2 1

To all the Air Evac nurses whom I have had the wonderful opportunity to have known and worked with. They are truly the top guns of the nursing ladder. The world is a better place because of their dedication to nursing.

And most of all, to Pam Childress, for without her encouragement, dedication, and sacrifice, this book would never have been written.

I rhythmically moved my flattened palms up and down on his chest, praying that the very desire bashing the insides of my ribcage could be forced from my body into his by the sheer strength of my need for him to live. "God . . . damn . . . you . . . " The words spewed from my mind, only to be trapped in the constriction of my throat, never to be heard by those men and women surrounding me. "Don't you dare die! I won't let you! I won't! I won't!"

I don't know why it so surprised me that my mind had suddenly started working on two levels. While I automatically measured the depth and timing of the chest compressions, I, at once, watched it all in a state of limbo. God help me, I didn't want the young man below me to die. I wanted, desperately needed, to see him smile, hear him laugh, watch him live. He wouldn't. And I, after ten challenging and fulfilling years of caring for the critically ill, after even more years in which I taught nursing, and three great wonder-filled years of being an Air Evac nurse, I died with Airman John Sloane. Thousands of miles from nowhere, on the farthest island of the Alaskan chain, it was over. For both of us.

I sucked air between my lips and pressed my front teeth hard in on themselves. John Sloane had transferred to the Air Force base on Shimea a week earlier. It didn't seem long enough for something to happen to take his life. It was a tragic and unfortunate accident, and totally unfair.

As he lay there, so young, so still—so dead—a sensation of intense desolation swept over me. The bitterness of cold despair crept into the very corners of my soul and lay there, a festering wound robbing me of all power. I closed my eyes, willing away the aching torment that had locked its unforgiving grip on my heart. I was a nurse. I had to handle this, as I had done hundreds of times before.

I tried. I had desperately tried to help save John Sloane, and couldn't.

Outside the dark caves of my mind I heard Elise gently coaxing the others into going through the steps necessary to close the book on Airman Sloane. My mind closed, too. I knew that as the charge nurse my job was no longer to remain with the patient but to make other preparations. I had to deal with that.

Elise prodded me toward the door, telling me to go to work on the reams of paperwork the government required for everything, even death. She was a saint in a flight suit. She knew somehow I needed to get out of that room.

I left the room and stepped outside into the cold morning with darkness all around me except for the dull light glimmering through the door out of which I had just stepped. I was so thankful to be able to leave that room that an involuntary shiver racked my body. I tilted my face to the dark, clear, cold sky. Taking a deep breath and trying to hold back the tears, I stood there thinking back to why I was where I was. What was it that made me want to fly Air Evac so badly?

Contents

Preface

Every day, for most of my adult life, I made the difference between pain and comfort, fear and tranquility, life and death. It was a power not to be taken lightly. Real people, not just names on a well-scribbled chart, but mothers, fathers, brothers, and sisters, placed their lives in my hands. They did it with hope, with faith, and with an intense need to be made whole again. They, and everyone who loved them, trusted me.

I wouldn't let them down.

I'm a nurse.

ANGEL WINGS

One
The Beginning

Muted shafts of sunlight filtered through the practical venetian blinds curtaining a long row of windows in the cafeteria. As usual, my friend Mary had let herself become distracted by the small slices of grass and trees visible through the slats.

"So," she let the word deflate on a cushion of expelled air, "how does the new crop of students look?"

I smiled. Mary was the charge nurse of the medical floor at the local military hospital our school used for its clinical training site. An active duty Air Force nurse, she was good—one of those people truly gifted with the intuition and intelligence to be exceptional in the field. I loved bringing students from the small, private nursing school where I taught for new insights. She always gave them more than I could have possibly wanted.

"Great," I said, "I really love teaching, and I think a number of them have a lot of potential."

Mary made a face, one I'd come to know as her "yes, but" preamble, and punched her half-empty glass with a brightly striped straw. "Isn't there anything else you've ever wanted to do, though? I mean, other than teaching, or maybe in addition to it. I don't know, I was just thinking that maybe you'd like to try something else."

"What's up, Mary?"

"Up?" Soft blue eyes penetrated deep into mine. We'd

known each other long enough and worked together often enough that keeping professional secrets was possible, but not probable.

I sighed. "I've worked some pretty tough assignments, Mary. I left critical care to teach to protect myself from serious burnout. It's what I do now, and I consider it a very important job."

"Number one," Mary tapped a short, well-buffed nail on the table, "all nursing jobs are important. Number two, I know something you don't."

"What?" We'd spent a lot of hours together talking about life, love, happiness, and the sometimes overwhelming stress of nursing.

But this time, Mary had a positively wicked gleam in her eye. She'd obviously thought about whatever she had in mind for me, and I wasn't at all sure I had a chance against her. From the very first moment I laid eyes on her, I liked the pretty blonde who so deftly handled what to most people would have been a difficult job. Mary was one of the few charge nurses I knew who had managed to circumvent the Peter Principle.

The Peter Principle. What a pain (no pun intended!) it could become on a nursing ward! It worked simply and, sadly, frequently, to wreak havoc amongst otherwise dedicated colleagues. It's really just a matter of bureaucracy. They take a nurse who knows what she's doing, knows the ins and outs of patient care, does her job especially well. She performs well, so they promote her until she is no longer in charge of bedside patient care, the very thing that she did so well. Instead, she's in charge of other nurses who are in charge of direct patient care. She has become a charge nurse. This continues to happen. A nurse performs well and she is promoted. If she continues to perform well, she's promoted again. Sooner or later, she reaches a level where she no longer performs competently. And as often as not, she's miserable in her job and makes life miserable for those who are around her. The Peter Principle—a la Florence Nightingale.

But Mary was different. She was well suited to be the charge nurse. She was also well suited to getting me involved in exciting and far-flung adventures.

"Lori," she smiled sweetly, "I went to the Philippines."

My ears perked up. Ah, travel. How I wanted to go places, have money to spend, meet great men, and have a chance to challenge my nursing. This could be it. Mary had been an Air Evac flight nurse with the military, flying to such places as Guam, Germany, France, Korea, and more—all the places I so craved seeing. I'd often fantasized about those places and the exciting life she'd led, imagining it as my own. Still, at the moment, I was more interested in the cause for Mary's sweet smile and totally unexpected announcement that she'd been to the Philippines, or PI as she refers to it. Something was up, and to be honest, I could barely wait to find out what.

"Okay, you have my attention." I knew I had to bite. Mary hadn't brought up the subject of my teaching and her trip to the PI for no reason. "What do the PI and my job have in common?"

Mary stared out the window, all innocence and light. "Nothing, Lori. Why, nothing at all." Blue eyes turned on me. "Want to go to a party this Saturday?"

I was in deep trouble. This tiny little pack of dynamite I called my friend had just mumbled less than a dozen words that were about to change my life completely.

I guess the time was ripe for changes in my life. I was teaching nursing, after leaving my career in critical care. It had been a long journey, my stint of caring for the patients in the worst condition at McBride Hospital. While it was an extraordinarily gratifying job, it was also one that tended to require off time. I'd put in ten years—more than most nurses who enter the critical care field—and found myself needing a lighter load with less pressure. Many people think nurses can just "turn it off" and not get involved in the pain and heartache surrounding their patients. While, for professional reasons, we must sometimes function as if that was the case, in actuality we're an extremely empathetic group. People who don't care about other people just don't become nurses. Oh, sure, there are those who like the uniform, like the relative job security, or are looking for a doctor to marry. But few of them last, and I wasn't one of them.

Instead I spent years in nursing, practicing my craft and helping those with the most critical need. Eventually, fearing burnout, I obtained my master's degree and went into teaching. I'd reached a point in my life where I needed to get away from the sickness and pursue some of the dreams I had before I'd dedicated myself to critical care.

When I was a teenager, I'd known two things for certain: one, I wanted to own and raise thoroughbred horses, the other, that I was going to fly. I longed to climb aboard one of the huge, powerful planes and jet around the world—shopping the myriad marketplaces of Germany, partying in exotic Hawaiian nightclubs, running on the sun-drenched beaches of Guam, and jumping horses over monolithic downed trees in Alaska. Unlike so many people who spent their lives wondering what they really want, I was blessed. I knew, completely and fervently, what I wanted my past, present, and future to hold. I just didn't know what a fantastic journey I would undertake to get there. And I didn't know how much of it was going to come about as the result of a seemingly innocuous remark made over an iced Coke in a nondescript cafeteria!

Sometimes things camouflage themselves as something else. That was Mary. She thought she was an Air Force charge nurse. What she really was was an angel, a fair-haired courier of wonderful things. She didn't realize it. Nor did she plot it or even, for that matter, bring it in any expected sort of way. What she did was, quite simply, plop a magic sphere at my feet. To her it was just a party, one she had good reason to believe I would enjoy, perhaps even find adventurous. But just a party, nonetheless.

To this day, I truly believe, though, that she felt a need to introduce me to the world of Air Force nursing. She knew I found my work as an army reservist training medics at the Presidio Army Base in San Francisco exciting and challenging. She also knew that I craved more. Realizing these things, she thought I would enjoy the annual 25th Air Evac Christmas party. To her it was a chance for me to meet new people involved in a different type of medicine, one that was practiced at forty thousand feet. If she thought I would be excited by all that, she was right!

It was an hour's drive to Tently Air Base. During the drive Mary and I had ample time to talk, and talk we did. Mary wove wonderful stories about her experiences as a flight nurse. All the time her eyes sparkled and a faint glow suffused her tanned skin.

"I remember when I was stationed in the Philippines," she began. (*Ah, at last,* I thought, *the connection.*) "One of the missions we'd fly was to Alaska." Mary settled back in her seat, the road to Tently so well known to her that she could dedicate herself fully to the memory. "When we got there, we were left to our own to find a way back to the Philippines."

"Didn't they take you back?" I questioned. It seemed

odd to me that the Air Force would make a habit of stranding its personnel on remote—and decidedly cold—corners of the world.

Mary's nose scrunched into a wrinkle. "Of course. I mean, well, for example one plane came in, from the PI, and was headed to the lower forty-eight, . . . Idaho, I think. Anyway, I was left to find my own way back to PI. I was allowed to hitch a ride on any one of our planes headed in that direction, but this time there weren't any until the next day. So I went to the bachelor officers' quarters, or BOQ, to get a room only to find that they were full."

"So you were stuck, weren't you?" I was beginning to wonder about this "great job" Mary was always telling me about. Why would anyone be so thrilled about an occupation that entailed being stranded in Alaska without a place to stay?

"No. Do you want to hear this story or not?" She scolded in what must have been her best you're-being-difficult voice.

"Yes, yes, continue." I tried to sound reticent, but I'm afraid she knew I wasn't frightened.

"You're incorrigible, Lori," Mary laughed. "But I'll turn you on to Air Evac nursing yet!"

I couldn't help but laugh with her. "Go on, tell me more, I'll shut up."

"To make a long story short, more or less, there were also nine pilots who were looking for a place to spend the night at the same time I was. They suggested we all sleep in the dayroom."

I tried, unsuccessfully, I'm afraid, to keep my eyes from becoming saucers. I knew what a dayroom was. Just one large room with couches and tables, it was more of an oversized, underdecorated living room than a place where one woman and nine men could spend the night. I never thought I had that active an imagination, but at the moment, I was looking at Mary from a whole different point of view.

"Now, knock that off!" Mary burst into a flurry of nervous giggles. "Nothing happened like that, but a lot of other things did."

I raised a brow. I couldn't help it. Mary was my friend, but . . . nine men?

"Truly, Lori," Mary worked to get the laughter under control, "You wouldn't believe it. It was twelve midnight, and we were all tired. Still, I kind of balked at the idea, but I was too beat to try to work out anything else, so I just went along. And believe it or not, it was great. They all just sort of took me under their wing and laid out some cushions on the floor. They even dug up a blanket and tucked me in just like I was a favorite sister or something. We all talked for awhile, sharing stories about who we were and where we were from and all. Next thing I knew, I was waking up. It was six-thirty in the morning, and everyone was slowly gathering their things and leaving to catch planes to wherever they were going."

Mary smiled. It was a pleasant memory, one that she relished reliving. That much was evident in the contentment in her voice, the softness in her eyes.

"Lori, can you imagine how really nice it is to have nine men take care of you with such gentleness? Not one of them tried to put the make on me or even insinuated that because I was a woman, I could be less than, or maybe just different from, a friend. The military is great for that. Friends."

Mary sighed, and I, well, I guess if I'm to be honest, I was falling in love. With the Air Force, with Air Evac nursing, with my old dreams of flying, and with this wonderful new nursing challenge.

By the time we got to the gate at Tently, I could feel a nervous tingling building inside my stomach. I couldn't help asking myself, am I really doing this? And most important, will it ever culminate in the high drama of flight nursing, shopping in exotic places, seeing the world, and meeting new and exciting friends? Best yet, reaching into a whole new arena with my nursing? Finding and experiencing the opportunity to delve into my profession as few people ever can?

It was definitely an enticing possibility. I'd always thrived on new challenges in medicine and, particularly now, felt a deep need to move on to yet another frontier. Beyond that was the inevitable knowledge that I had reached the point where I vested far too much of my personal emotions in my patients. Increasingly I found myself feeling responsibility toward them far beyond what was humanly and medically possible to deliver. This has always been a problem in the nursing profession and, as much as all of us in the field think we will be immune, it catches up to us in the long run. It caught up to me. And I was too much of a professional not to take it seriously.

I needed new horizons. I needed new challenges. To be frank, I needed to distance myself from ICU and I hoped Air Evac would do it.

There was something else, something very tangible and very important. When I first began to realize I was facing the all too real possibility of burnout, I made a conscious decision not to leave nursing altogether as some men and women do. The job was too important to me and, I felt, too important to society to disclaim. I made no apologies then, and I make none now, for this position. There are those who would consider such a comment pompous, but I have only one thing to say to those people: When you are in a field of service as vital as caring for the health and lives of others, it's a sad and wasteful thing to let your knowledge and experience go to waste. There are too few nurses. Losing one can, and does, make a difference. Not that I'm proposing that we're irreplaceable. We aren't. Yet, there are too few willing to take our place. This left me with only two alternatives: one, to continue in ICU and risk the physiologic, psychologic, and social stress associated with the profession; or two, to look into new types of nursing.

So it was that I found myself propelled toward the horizon.

The setting sun was casting a warm amber glow over the countryside by the time we reached the gate at Tently Air Force Base. But for once, Mother Nature hadn't managed to outshine mortal man. I entered an entirely different world when I stepped through the door of the Air Evac building.

In the multipurpose room (for lack of a better word), one of the most imaginative parties I've ever seen had been laid out. It was an extraordinarily provocative scene, not as the result of decorations or any type of predetermined ambience, but rather by the sheer force of the personalities gathered there. And I don't mean provocative in a sexual sense, although there were more than enough handsome men in that overburdened room to make any woman's blood run hot. The whole situation was just . . . impressive.

To call the people of the 25th eclectic is an understatement along the lines of calling rocks hard. The women were clothed in everything from evening gowns to Levis and imprinted sweatshirts. A devastatingly gorgeous brunette leaned against one wall in what I was sure was a Nolan Miller gown replete with his trademark bugle beading. The dress could have easily cost as much as some people's cars. Her hair was a perfect example of Jose Eber's "shake your head, darling" platitudes; it looked as if it was moving in a gentle breeze, even though, on careful examination, it obviously wasn't.

Not ten feet from her, the tallest, thinnest redhead I'd ever seen was wearing tight Levis 501s under an oversized T-shirt adamantly proclaiming "Property of Yale Athletic Department." The redhead had draped herself on the arm of a beribboned full-dress colonel. You could have done your makeup in the glossy reflections of his perfectly polished shoes.

I expected Allen Funt to jump from behind the somewhat withered ficus and scream, "Smile!" When it became obvious that he wouldn't, I gave up and turned my attention to Rich, the bartender, who, by the way, was very worthy of heaping attention on.

Mary and I headed straight for the bar upon our arrival. Carrying a cocktail, whether you drank it or not, seemed almost sacrosanct at this party. Mary opted for an iced orange juice. I wanted a simple white wine and a not-so-simple cute bartender. From the looks of him, Rich had been born for the sole purpose of charming women. If it hadn't have been for Mary's dragging me away to meet some of her friends, he could have quickly absorbed me with those mischievous eyes and sweet smiles.

He was interesting. It seemed that everyone there was interesting. When I focused on the women Mary was introducing me to, I realized how rarely a person would ever see so many beautiful, well-dressed, intelligent nurses congregated in such a small area. The list of advanced degrees and impressive job titles—administrator, director, manager, to name but a few—were inspiring. As someone who knew the time and commitment as well as the intelligence and savvy necessary to earn what these women had achieved, I was truly impressed. My mind began clicking. Mary had spent the evening introducing me as her Army friend, always following it with the refrain that she intended to convert me to an Air Force nurse from the 25th.

It sounded good to me! And it was sounding better and better by the minute. Ironically, part of the appeal came from some rather unexpected sources. As Mary and I were making the rounds of the room, I was surprised to find so many people I knew from hospitals I had worked at before. It was funny how seeing someone you know who was once in the same position as you and had grown more successful whets your appetite to do the same.

Some of my old friends from McBride, a hospital I'd worked at several years before, were at the party. Some old gossip mates, some old boyfriends. . . .

Like Boomer. Oh, boy, Boomer. What can one say about Boomer Jones? That he was a clever, fun-loving man with a thatch of thick hair that just begged to be handled? That you never knew up from down, in from out, when he was around? That I always thought he should be married—to anyone except me?

I'd dated him when I first arrived in Sacramento. At the time, he was an orderly at McBride Hospital, where I was an intensive care nurse. He was smart. In fact, it was obvious to me that Boomer was an extremely intelligent man. Problem was, it seemed no one had ever bothered to let Boomer in on how bright he was. Well, no. That's not true. What I should say is that no one ever made him understand the good, the bad, and the ugly of his mind. Boomer had always come across as a know-it-all, which was all the more irritating because he generally was. The problem was that he never really put all that brain power to good use. Instead, I always felt as if we were involved in some sort of competitive race, one in which I had absolutely no idea where he'd set the finish line. We had some great times together, but I eventually got bored with his antics.

I was really thrilled to meet his new wife. It was nice to see someone else at his side. That, more than anything else, I guess, provided the deepest insight into our past relationship.

It seemed that the 25th had been a good drawing card for former McBride staff. Just as I was making my good-byes to Mr. and Mrs. Boomer Jones, I spotted another McBride alumnus. The recovery room nurse who had worked the same weekend shifts as I was standing not more than three feet away, dressed to the teeth, as was her wont.

Virginia Starr had been and still was beautiful, efficient, beautiful, ambitious, beautiful, intelligent, and beautiful. She was also, at least at the moment, doing a fantastic imitation of a snob. We'd known each other for years, but she very deftly pushed aside my hello by pretending she didn't know who I was. I knew I'd changed, but since I hadn't had plastic surgery, dyed my blonde hair brown, gained or lost a hundred pounds or grown a second head, I expected that she would remember me. She very obviously didn't. Too obviously, in fact.

That was one of my first glimpses into the working of the Starr mind. I didn't know yet how frightened I should have been. Instead, I felt a little offended, but not enough to keep me from wondering if she was still married to the doctor from McBride she'd become engaged to while I was there. Virginia had made a lovely bride-to-be; so lovely, in fact, that she kept repeating her performance.

In those days, it didn't take much to draw my attention away from the illustrious Ms. Starr (a habit self-preservation soon forced me to break!).

The crowd was rapidly getting thicker, and the party was definitely started. Even though I'd dallied maybe a little longer than normal picking up my second drink from the bar (blame it on that low, silvery voice and poetic flattery), it wasn't long before I found myself holding court on the edge of the crowd. Remember when you were fifteen and there was nothing more exciting than to be surrounded by cute guys dangling on your every word? That's holding court, and let me tell you, it's twice as great when you're thirty-eight! Flattery and attention, I think, are far, far underrated as innocent pastimes. The people gathered for the 25th Air Evac Christmas party more than proved my point; we were all there for one reason and one reason only—it was Christmas and we wanted to have some company; we wanted to have some fun.

It was like something out of a movie. All the men were handsome in their flight suits and dress uniforms, even those in civilian clothes had the unmistakable aura of men who fly. Whether they were captains, majors, lieutenant colonels, or something else, they all had the same thing in common; they worked in the sky. There was an almost tangible pride in that room. It was evident in the way the men laughed, in the teasing curves of the women's lips. It didn't matter whether their teeth were perfect or in need of braces. Everyone that night had Pepsodent smiles. It was almost magic.

Mary laid her palm on my arm and pointed toward a small stage that had been set up on the far side of the room. Simultaneously, over two hundred sets of eyes turned toward the planking that was suddenly bathed in light. I could hardly believe the new shape of insanity that was forming there. A positively irreverent take-off of "Saturday Night Live" was happening before my eyes!

These people really were a let's-pull-out-all-the-stops-and-be-goofy bunch. A flight nurse attired head to toe in what could have only been a 1950s telephone operator's castoffs simpered and snorted her way across stage and unceremoniously dumped her hunch-shouldered body on a chair facing the audience.

Mary giggled. "God! Where on earth did she get that outfit? She looks just like Lily Tomlin!"

Before I had the chance to even try to find my voice, the music stopped and the room was filled with the booming command, "Ladies, gentlemen, whoever, the skit is about to begin."

"What skit?" I craned my neck trying to see and was immediately rewarded by a man standing just in front of me with a gentle nudge toward a better view.

"Every year they have these skits," Mary raised her voice to be heard above the din of the crowd. "They're always funny and have to do with Air Evac."

A young, tough-looking medical technician swaggered up to the woman on the stage. His muscles rippled, his mouth curled in a positively lewd leer, and the crowd went wild. Not even Stallone could have put on a more potent display of egotistical machismo than this guy. Immediately sliding into a satirical vein, the nurse whined dumb comments in a nasal voice while the med-tech flexed and dominated. It was a great send-up, mocking the reality of Air Evac, where nurses are all officers and in control and med-techs are usually male enlisted personnel charged with doing the physical work.

Part of the skit included a video tape of a tech who became hypoxic and consequently confused and disoriented during flight. Hypoxia happens when you can't breathe due to lack of oxygen, and although it can be frightening and deadly, it can also be extremely funny.

Someone suffering from hypoxia the way the med-tech was in the skit will say and do absolutely outrageous things. Later, the same person might not even remember what he did or said. The skit was very clever and offered an insightful, albeit hysterical, view from the inside of Air Evac.

As the skit reined to a close, a simulation of an Air Evac mission including the tricks and tribulations of the trade was presented. Gripping Murphy's Law around the throat, the scriptwriter employed its full effect and put those poor actors through everything from miscommunication at the outset to a potentially lethal plane crash at the end. And what was the result? Well, it *was* Air Evac doing the skit; the beautiful blue-eyed blonde (her too-perfect body I don't even want to try to describe!) "patient" was able to jump up from her stretcher and walk away unscathed.

Due entirely to the great training and unerring dedication of the Air Evac nurses and medical technicians, she had been saved. Unfortunately, everyone else died. Oh, well, nobody's perfect, and the show was well done.

By the time the skit ended, so many more people had poured into the building, it was bursting at the seams. I was getting ready to get myself another drink (Rich was, after all, still tending bar), when I felt some motion over my shoulder.

"May I buy you a drink?" The man behind me had a voice that was low, sensual, and making more than one nerve in my body tingle.

"Thank you, but that isn't necessary." His hair was blonde, his eyes were blue, and I was totally unable to stop staring at him and wishing he'd whisper in my ear again. Fortunately, he didn't believe a word I'd said.

His brows wrinkled over those killer cornflower blue

eyes for a second before he spoke again.

"I'm sorry. I guess I've done this wrong. My name is Ted. I'm a lieutenant colonel in charge of an engineering unit here at Tently, but most of the time I'm a lawyer. My practice is in San Francisco. If you're ever in trouble with the law," he smiled, deathly concerned with his next comment, "or very thirsty, I'd love to help you out."

"Okay," I couldn't help but laugh. "Since you put it that way, I'll take a white wine. And thank you."

Ted slipped into the space next to me. "You're welcome, umm, pretty blonde lady who forgot to give me her name."

"Lori Drew." I slipped my hand out, expecting him to take it. He did. Thing was, he didn't give it back. Not that I cared, mind you. "I teach nursing in Sacramento. I'm also an army reservist stationed out of the Presidio. I used to race horses, and I just decided I love blue eyes."

"Well, since I have blue eyes, I think that maybe we should find a place to sit and talk. We evidently have a lot in common."

Ted was totally charming. He had one of the cutest smiles I had ever seen, and he was obviously a talented and successful man. We had a wonderful time, one moment discussing important topics, the next making small talk. I was comfortable with him, something that doesn't always happen with someone you've just met. It was a bit disappointing when Mary came over to tell me it was time to leave. But I was already past drunk and lunging headfirst toward completely soused, so I just gave Ted my phone number and amenably followed Mary out the door. It had been a great evening; my mind was soaring with new ideas, new hopes, and renewed dreams.

As it turned out, Ted and I saw each other again a week later, but it didn't work out. When all the glory and festivities had dwindled to a one-on-one relationship, it came down to Ted being a great guy, but not for me. I never saw him again after that. But it was the beginning of a whole new adventure for me. That night at the 25th Christmas bash, I decided I wanted to join that squadron.

Two
Taking the Step

At thirty-eight years old and single, I knew this was the time to do it. Instinct told me to stop thinking and dreaming and just go ahead and reach for the pinnacle. Air Evac offered the chance to experience a different type of nursing, one that would require all of my skills and knowledge in a new and unstable environment. I would have to push myself to the limit of my knowledge. I would also be able to travel, make some money, and take part in fantastic adventures. Air Evac would be the greatest challenge of my career!

Still, it was a big step and a huge commitment, not only in time, but in physical and emotional energy as well. I wanted it. Oh, how I wanted it! But I also knew that though I craved a change in my life, actually going through it could be extremely stressful. One of the reasons I'd quit intensive care nursing and gone into teaching was to get away from keeping sick patients alive in the worst possible situations. Was this the same? Yes, but I could smell the challenge as if it were a tangible thing.

For two solid months I juggled with the problem. Finally, after forcing myself to reach deep inside and honestly look at motivation, I knew that I was going to go for it. It was my dream, and I knew in my heart of hearts that dreams were far too precious to throw away. Too often we lose ourselves just getting along with life when we could be soaring with passions.

I was going to do my damnedest to soar!

Unfortunately, wanting to be in the 25th and actually joining were two entirely different matters. The military wasn't like the Girl Scouts. You didn't just decide to "join up" and walk in and do it, especially since the branch and program I wanted to be in was somewhat of an elitist organization. Besides all the problems surrounding the Air Force, there was the Army to be dealt with. My tour with them wasn't yet finished, so I had to also convince my National Guard superiors to transfer my commission.

I really liked being part of the Army Guard, but it didn't offer me the opportunities to travel that I would have as an Air Evac nurse. So I had to sit down and really think out what I was going to do. One thing I've carried with me throughout all of my life is an undying belief that if you wanted something badly enough, no obstacle is too great to prevent you from getting it. At this point I wanted to join the Air Force Reserve; my belief in "if you want it, you'll get it" was going to be sorely tested before I made my dream come true.

The first, and perhaps most predictable, obstacle was just getting my commission transferred. I was an Army captain at the time and didn't relish losing my rank upon transferring to another service branch. However, I did have a master's degree in nursing. I knew that my education would carry some weight in that department. First I tried to see if I could stay in the National Guard, but was told that that would be impossible. That left leaving the Guard and going to the Air Force my only alternative. Sadly, the Army National Guard wasn't really happy about releasing me.

In order to be dropped honorably from the Guard, I had to convince my commander and chief nurse to write a letter to the Air Force saying that they would release me. They hesitated, thinking that I wasn't serious about wanting out.

There had been a time while I was in the Guard that I'd gotten involved in a relationship with one of the pilots. My chief nurse thought I was trying to run away from what had become a painful and disillusioning breakup. Maybe in some way I was. I don't know. I felt as if I was motivated by no more than a desire to be involved with an exciting new facet of nursing. Yes, I was eager to put the pilot behind me. Yes, leaving the Guard was almost guaranteeing that I would be far enough away not to be susceptible to falling back into a no-win relationship again. And yes, I wished more than ever to leave him far, far behind me, emotionally, mentally, physically.

Still, I remember vividly the excitement that ran through me when I received word from the Air Force that I'd been accepted in the Air Evac program. I was on cloud nine! Being accepted in and of itself was an incredible honor. The extensive applications I filled out, the ten-year-long list of job experience, extracurricular activities, letters of commendation, a mandatory security clearance, even proof of my earlier divorce had all to be formed, filed, and verified. It was obvious that not everyone who wanted to be in Air Evac was going to make it. Now, it seemed only two things stood in my way, both of them my commanding officers.

I went to my chief nurse's office after months had passed and no letter recommending my release had been forthcoming. I'm not a restless person, but I found myself almost fidgeting as I sat across her desk, waiting for the interview to begin. I couldn't decide whether to be concerned that no matter what I might say she wouldn't let me go or to be angry that she hadn't already let me go.

Before any single emotion could gel, I had to ask her permission to do what I wanted with my life. (This is one facet of the military that I never really came to grips with.)

"You know," I said, "I really would like to join the Air Force."

Instead of the abrupt no I'd expected, the chief nurse looked a bit confused. "But why? I thought you'd forgotten all about that."

"No. No." I leaned forward in my chair, an excited tingling building in my head. "I really do want to go over to the Air Force. It's not that I don't like the Guard. I do. But ever since I was a little girl, I've wanted to fly. I tried to become a stewardess, but because of a kidney problem, couldn't. I'm thirty-eight years old and I really need to do this. I need to fulfill my dream of flying. And I can do that there, but not here."

"Well," she laced her hands under her chin, "what about this pilot you've been having a personal problem with?"

"I want to fly Air Evac. I want to meet the challenge."

She watched me for a few seconds, seemingly digesting everything. In the long run, I think it was my choice to simply state my desire to fly rather than defend my love life that won her over. At any rate, she relented and wrote the letter. After an almost identical (do they have a script for these things?) conversation with my commander, the second, and final, letter went out. I was no longer an Army Guard Captain.

All that was left between me and the cloud-filled sky was the Big Physical. If ever a thing deserved to be written in capital letters this physical did! I'd been a nurse for years and was still overwhelmed by it, more than anything, because I knew that my history of kidney problems could rear its ugly head and ground me before I even took off. I asked my doctor for verification that the hydronephrosis had been corrected. Since he was able to confirm it, that was taken care of, but there was always the possibility that I'd fail the actual physical.

The Big P. Ouch. If you have a hole they check it. If you have a quiver they shake it. If you have a button they push it. And if every tooth, bump, curve, and slope isn't functioning just right, they give you a pink slip and send you back to the farm. I was scared. I was praying. Then I was relieved—I passed!

I was on my way!

So much time had passed between when I first decided to try Air Evac and when I actually reported for flight school that I had plenty of time to reconcile any difficulties I might have had. This is easier said now than it was done then, but consider the timetable I was working with. It took two months just to get an application from the Air Force so that I could request being considered for the program. It was complex and extensive to the point that it took a month to fill it out. It always took six months to a year from the time of submission to acceptance, providing you were accepted. Once you were admitted, you were sworn in and assigned. Only after you received an assignment (mine was Tently AFB just out of Sacramento, California) were you scheduled for flight school. When I went in, it took another eight months from the date of assignment to the squadron until reporting to flight school. I hear it's only four months now. An improvement, I think.

I was breathing easier by then. I had, after all, already hurdled quite a few major obstacles, as well as my release from the Army Guard and my kidney stones, I was well past thirty-three, the maximum age limit set for women who want to enter Air Evac nursing. From what I heard, it was only because of my outstanding National Guard record, extensive education, and three years in the reserves and Medivac training that they agreed to make an exception to my age. All I had to do from then on was show the 25th I could be an Air Evac nurse. And wait. And work.

I trained medics for the Army Guard at the Presidio clear up through the first month that I reported to the Air Force. I definitely missed the medics I was training in the emergency room. It was really hard to give up that part of my life. Harder than I'd expected. Real hard. But I did.

And then it was time to report to the first day of Air Evac . Now there was an enlightening experience. Going from the Army to the Air Force, was a whole different ball game. It was as different as apples from oranges.

One would think that two different branches of the same government entity would be fairly consistent with each other regarding lifestyles, expectations, etcetera. They are, one could argue, both under the umbrella of the Department of Defense, both an organization of soldiers and complementary personnel, both serving the same purpose, if not destined to perform the same job. All of that is true. But it's more involved than that in actuality.

You see, the Army is the Army. It's the military, and that's exactly how they see themselves. The troops in green. The Air Force is a support branch of the Army, and their whole way of thinking is totally different than the Army.

When you're in the Army, you quickly learn that they have a way of saying, "We want you to look good, but are you functional, too?"

They don't really put much store in the creature comforts. If you're given a room by billeting, it would probably be something out of an old John Wayne movie, with wood floors, a cot, maybe a chair, and a tiny towel. Even the showers lacked grace; they perpetually ran cold. But in the Air Force, there is a definite emphasis on looking good. You are expected to be well turned *and* well trained. They cared about the creature comforts in a way that startled me.

I'll never get over my first brush with this mind-set. My first, and each subsequent, Air Force room came with a radio, my own closet, a (hot!) shower, comfortable bed, rugs, and a color TV. There was even alcohol in my room. I mean, it was a different, totally different world. I felt as if I'd fallen from an austere compartment into the lap of luxury.

I have to confess, though, that I felt the Air Force put the emphasis in the wrong place. I mean, what was the difference whether my buckles were shined or not? How could that help me to perform better? Sometimes the unending spit and polish would get to me, but that's what they wanted, and so, those were the things I had to deal with on a day-to-day basis. At least they were consistent—everyone from top brass on down had to be bright and shiny.

The last time I had a reprieve from the constant polish and press was the first day I reported. On that day I arrived in civilian clothes, just as everyone else had. There were six of us who reported at the same time. Little did I know at the time how incredibly important those five people would be in my life. Some of them were to become lasting friends. Some were destined to be a lasting influence on my perceptions, not only of my own private world, but of the larger portrait that is mankind as a whole.

One woman immediately stood out from the others in our small group. Her name was Mila Jones-Smith. She liked being a hyphenate. To her it was a special badge of womanhood to keep her last name attached to her maiden name in that way. I don't think she did it from a strong feminist consciousness or even a streak of liberalism as much from feeling a proprietary air about both names. They were hers. I had the feeling that very little else was hers with any permanency. Sadly, I was proven right.

Mila had no prior service, and I felt almost an obligation to take her under my wing. It wasn't an unwanted obligation, though. I liked her immediately. She was special, but no one would have thought so from outward appearances. She looked frail and kind of pathetic standing there amongst all those robust, outdoorsy types. She had barely squeaked into Air Evac under the age limit, having celebrated her thirty-second birthday, not yet reaching the big three-three.

Mila looked very pale and sickly the day I met her, to the point of seeming capable of being easily overwhelmed by the situation. That she didn't feel well that day was the only reason she seemed forlorn and plain. Once I got to know her, I discovered a dynamo, albeit a different sort of one. She gave the impression one could run right over her and hear not a whimper. No wonder everyone was surprised when she turned out to be an extremely competent and assertive home health care nurse with a long list of impressive recommendations.

Nonetheless, Mila had no idea what she'd gotten into. There she was, surrounded by eager and excited professionals and all she wanted to do was rest her sick body and tired mind. I was a captain and had military experience, so I did my best to help her through the endless lists of must-dos, must-not-dos, and take-care-of-its. I didn't know then how really sick she was. It only became evident when she didn't show up the next day.

But then, there was the rest of the bunch. A bunch of bananas is what! Ginger. Judy. Lynne. Bert. Talk about a rowdy group of people. No wonder poor Mila was such a lost sheep that first day. Some witch doctor must have thrown a voodoo spell over our spirits as we stepped into line. Our personalities harmonized and coincided with each other so perfectly, we could sometimes get into a rhythm that made our highjinks look like a cleverly choreographed dance. We ran rings around everybody. Before long, rumor around the base was that we were one of the most intelligent, tuned in, and assertive groups they'd ever had. Rumor held true.

What most other groups would normally accept, we'd balk at and refuse to do. We challenged everything. We questioned everything. Our byword quickly became "Why?"

"Do this." A pained smile from someone desperately trying to make us toe the line.

"Why?" Someone inevitably chimed.

"Always do this before that." They'd say.

"Why?" We'd reply.

"Never let such and such happen.

"Why?"

"Why?"

"Why?"

We were a pain in the ass, but we represented a new, outgoing personality, and before long they not only accepted it, but even encouraged it. I hadn't joined Air Evac to make changes, but when paired with the eclectic bunch of screw-looses chance had thrown together, I did. Air Evac equaled party time. New rule. Nobody bothered to ask why.

And as hard as we partied, twice that diligently we

worked. Always searching, always finding a better way to care for our patients. Always eager to give it our all, we were a unit with a goal. And we saw to it that our goals were met—and were exceeded—both professionally and personally.

Three
The Parties, the Pilots

They called us the Group. We liked to party a lot. We spent most of the time in the officer's club when we weren't in the unit. You know, all work and no play makes Lori, Ginger, Judy, Lynne, Bert, Mila (take your pick) a dull nurse.

We were the ones responsible for starting parties again between the pilot units and the Air Evac units. It was a venerable old tradition but had died out because there was a staleness in the unit in regard to mingling. The Group couldn't have that. After all, what's the point of being in the air force if you can't mingle with the fly boys?

The Christmas party had been great, and I was a bit disappointed to discover that day-to-day contact with all of those fun people was almost nonexistent. I broached the subject to the other nurses one night over dinner.

"Has anyone besides me ever been to one of the 25th's Christmas bashes?" I lanced a sweet and sour shrimp with my chopstick.

Ginger snatched it just before I could get it in my mouth. "Yeah. Did you go to the one last year?"

At least, that's what I think she said. It was a bit hard to understand her, considering how that shrimp, in addition to a positively huge chunk of eggroll, inflated her cheeks.

Mila eyed the other patrons in the crowded Chinese restaurant. She pursed her lips, pondered a moment, then opted not to be embarrassed by Ginger's faux pas. Ginger was Ginger. If you let her embarrass you, you spent far too much time red in the face.

"I did," Judy crowed. As usual, she caught on fast.

"Has anyone heard of any big blowouts coming off soon?" I tried to act innocent, even though I don't do innocent very well.

Bert crushed his wonton into a dusty heap. "I hear they don't do that stuff here anymore."

We all turned and eyed him suspiciously. "Why?" The Mormon Tabernacle Choir couldn't have sung it with more precision.

The Group had just entered into a pact to party. So we did.

The shocker was that we were actually encouraged to. I guess some bigwig somewhere thought it was good for PR. I didn't know why. To tell you the truth, I didn't much care. They definitely did nothing to stop us. That's what I cared about.

Right away, we began planning parties at the officer's club after our unit drills. We got some pretty good responses, which worked well to generate better relationships in the airplanes, too. As the theory goes, the family that plays together, stays together. We just took that one logical step further. If you had a good time with someone, you stopped looking at them as nothing more than another piece of machinery and began seeing them as a person. Soon we started to really know these men and women, and that was good. I'm proud of helping that to happen. It was no small trick. It turned out that besides having some fun, we did something that helped build good personal relationships and, consequently, smoother working conditions.

One problem lurked, though. It took a while for us to

go to flight school, and we weren't all going to get to go together. We all kind of went one at a time. It wasn't because of our roughhousing at Tently, but because of a flaw inherent in the training system.

There were only so many slots available to fit us into each six week course, and the courses were at eight-week intervals. The waiting was frustrating, but we tried to keep occupied. (Okay, so we didn't have much trouble in that area, we still got tired of waiting. Especially as each of us left and came back with outrageous and exciting stories about flight school.)

One of the things I did to pass the time was to run the immunization clinic. Actually, I jumped at the chance. It was fun and gave me a chance to meet a lot of people. Almost everyone in the Air Force had to get shots because we traveled all over the world and being current with immunizations was mandatory.

Because I'd been an educator, there were a lot of things I could teach the newer nurses at the clinic. I would come in and man the clinic, not only when I was regularly scheduled, but on my off weekends as well. Before long, I was getting pretty well known as the immunization nurse. It was enjoyable, and it gave me something else to do while I waited to go to flight school.

Because there wasn't much else we could do, the partying escalated as the weeks wore on. It reached the point where any time one of the Group met someone, they'd invite them to a party later that day or week.

I remember one time I met this officer who was a graduate of the Air Force Academy. Academy grads were considered the elite of the elite. It was hard to get into the academy and even harder to stay in. I was impressed. He was married. No great surprise.

Most of the pilots we met were married. After a while,

you stop looking to them for romantic relationships. A wedding band can strangle a lover faster than anything. Instead, we just tried to keep it light and entertaining. There's something to be said for just playing around without sexual entanglements or long-term commitments. You begin to look at the men you meet as someone to have fun with, because they're looking for something to do on the weekend while they're away from home and you want to party a little.

One part of the Air Force that is an aspect you quickly became acclimated to is that everybody you met was coming from or going all over the world, as well as all over the country. Any man or woman you were talking to could have been there merely because they were waiting for a flight out. Soon you began to expect one- and two-day friendships. It wasn't rough. In some ways it was actually invigorating and liberating. You can have fun unencumbered by tomorrows.

That's the way I looked at the academy grad I'd buddied up with. He was a NASA test pilot at that time and just starting his second childhood. I knew he had a son in the Air Force Academy and sometimes I wondered which one was youngest at heart. I suspected chronology had little to do with it. Quite a few times we climbed into his sports car and flew (he didn't realize you needed an airplane to go that fast) down to the river to picnic on a friend's boat. As many as ten of us would gather on the boat. A riot always broke loose with food and booze, singing and laughing—sometimes all day and all night.

The river is breathtaking. The sun had a way of roasting everyone to a deep golden hue, and we'd joke all day long, taking bets on who would come out with the best tan or worst burn. The terrain we boated through was wide open and opulent in its fertile fields. Onions, rice, and miles and miles of changing hues of brown and green would slip by in syncopated harmony. Everything looked different when viewed from the perspective of the water rather than the land. As I traveled more and more with the Air Evac, I discovered similar opposing views of earth's face applied also from the air.

Those long sunny days were a great outlet for me. I'd been running a nursing program, confining myself so much to Sacramento, I'd allowed my life to become a dull shadow of what it could be. I needed to have fun, take things a little less seriously when I wasn't actually working, and let my hair down now and then. The weekends with my Air Force friends opened up a whole new avenue I eagerly explored.

Sometimes we did nothing more than dance and sing at the officer's club all night, well until they closed. Other times we'd plan elaborate picnics and parties or converge on San Francisco like a swarm of hungry locusts. We would generate any scenario and live it out just to have fun. And it was good for me. It was good for all of us. Really good for all of us.

It was necessary, too. We all worked hard at our jobs, which we looked at as more than just jobs or careers, but as missions in life. We were dedicated almost to a man. As hard as we played, that much harder we worked.

Dig right in and take care of it could easily have been our motto. When you're a nurse you don't usually have much time to stop and decide, Do I really want to do this? Will it cost me too much physically, mentally, and emotionally? You do it. Period. And if one thing could be said for the nurses involved in Air Evac, it's that they were some of the most dedicated of them all.

Mila was like that. I remember so vividly the day she volunteered to work the clinic with me. When she came on duty, she looked even more tired and worn than usual, sort of like a well-used Raggedy Ann Doll. I knew she'd been working with a terminally ill patient for several weeks, staying long hours at his home to provide help and support to him and his family. This was Mila's nature. From her point of view, home health care meant she was a nurse not only to her actual patient, but also a friend and caring shoulder to the family as well.

No matter how often it happens—and in Mila's case, it was an inevitable conclusion of her medical specialty—the loss of a patient is hard. Sometimes, because of stress, illness, or other problems, it's even more difficult to come to grips with. And that's what had happened with John Anderson. He knew he was going to die, had been told at the outset. Mila, on the other hand, was secretly hoping for a miracle. There are a lot of miracles in medicine, but, unfortunately, John wasn't in line for one. So at almost noon the day before, he'd called Mila to his bedside. Death catches a lot of us by surprise, but once in awhile a patient seems to display an almost uncanny ability to read their own biological clock. John Anderson figured his was running out.

For a full forty minutes, he'd asked for nothing more than Mila to hold his hand. Then he turned his tired hazel eyes to her, whispered, "You made a difference," and fell asleep.

John Anderson never spoke again, and less than twelve hours later, Mila was standing in a brightly lit clinic giving shots to joking airmen. She seemed unaware of the incongruity of it all. But then, she was a nurse. You work. And you deal with it, as did we all.

I taught. I manned clinics. I trained. And before long, I was appointed public affairs officer to the unit. My stint as public affairs officer presented a great challenge to me.

One of the problems with the Air Force was that it had poor relations with the area newspapers. They only like to report the plane crashes and not any of the good stuff to people. This wasn't so uncommon, I suppose. The military ran on a different wave length—a different set of rules—than did civilians. The *Daily Gazette* was a civilian newspaper. I was going to make it my job to improve the rapport between the Air Force and the *Gazette*.

Luckily, I was able to network my way to victory in the Great *Gazette* Problem. A friend of a friend who was editor of the "Neighbors" section of the *Gazette* put out a good word and a subtle hint—"the women of Sacramento would love this story"—to those in power—you get my drift. Never underestimate the power of networking! Voilà. "Weekend Nurses in the Wild Blue Yonder" hit the presses on July 3, 1986. I was proud of myself for doing so well, but my success pissed off a few people. Like Virginia Starr.

Good old Virginia Starr. This broad was so self-centered, she expected Campbell's alphabet soup to spell her name as it was poured out of the can. She and I never really hit it off. The deliberate snub she had given me at the Christmas party was merely reflective of a basic personality flaw. It was too bad she hadn't decided then to ignore my existence forever. But with some things, I seem to have a streak of very bad luck. There were no leprechauns manning the trenches between me and the illustrious Virginia once the *Gazette* article hit the newsstands.

Basically, Virginia felt that she was the anointed one, Miss Air Evac 25th. Oh, yes, she was very attractive, very intelligent, and very talented. In fact, one of her talents was so finely tuned that she could have patented it. She called it moving up; I called it stabbing people in the back.

As Bert once observed, "It wouldn't surprise me if Old Lucky Starr has the word 'vindictive' tattooed on her ass."

I agreed. I would have looked except that the only people allowed to view the princess's derriere were men with sufficient rank to grant her power, money, or bennies.

The only thing predictable about Virginia was her unpredictability. She'd be smiling at you one minute and scratching your eyes out the next. This I found out too late. I'd already made the grave error of getting some attention for Air Evac and, by default, myself, with the *Gazette* story. Virginia ignored me from that moment on. This saddened me, not only because of the obvious problems on the job, but also because I had once admired her very much.

For the longest time I had really respected her. During the months prior to flight school, I tried to be friends with her and worked to develop a good relationship. It wasn't destined to happen. She would never let it. Because she was a damn good nurse, a lot of people looked up to her, but over the years she alienated almost everyone who spent much time with her. After awhile, we all, one by one, saw through Virginia and didn't want to be around her anymore. It was too bad she was the way she was. She truly was clever and talented enough to have climbed the ladder of success without the underhanded practices she employed. It was a waste. She could have had her cake and eaten it, too.

One of the things that was indicative of her unwarranted behavior occurred at the first Christmas party the 25th had after I joined. I'd been there only a couple of months and was looking forward to having everyone gathered in one place at one time. The parties the Group had generated were great, what with everything from baseball to barbecues to sourdough French bread bought fresh on Frisco's Fisherman's Wharf, but this promised to be great with a capital G.

The Group was pretty outspoken, and we all tended to show a lot of leadership. Those things can get you into a lot of trouble. They can also get you involved in some nice things as well. There were two nurses who put a lot of effort and affection in orienting us when we'd first arrived in Air Evac. We'd nicknamed them Mama Cherise and Grandma Betty. To show our appreciation for the job they did, we thought it would be nice to do a skit for them at the Christmas party. We went to work to put together a song and dialogue highlighting how well they'd succeeded in making us feel welcome, how they'd always been there when we needed them, and all the energy they'd used to get us through the processing to get us into the unit.

The party was in full swing, and we all had had more than one visit to the bar when we strutted on stage. The lights flashed, we hooted, the audience hollered, and all of us lined up like the Rockettes (as best we could, considering blood alcohol levels). I stepped a little ahead of the line, and we sang our song. Everyone seemed to be enjoying it, so we did a little dance and called Mama Cherise and Grandma Betty up on stage and presented each of them with a stuffed teddy bear. Mama Cherise actually started crying, and Grandma Betty was very, very touched. It made us feel so good to give some of the love back that they'd given to us.

It didn't make Virginia feel good, though. I could see her in the back; she made a pointed effort to pretend she wasn't watching our presentation. Virginia hated not being the center of attention. The jealousy literally radiated out of the back of her eyes. It almost made you sick to see her wanting to deny Cherise and Betty their small moment of glory. However, Virginia did get her award. The 25th honored her with a beautiful statue of a man and woman lying together kissing. A representation of the TDY award. The honor is bestowed on the person that had the most affairs during the year on TDY (temporary duty). Temporary duty is usually when you fly somewhere and stay overnight. Yes, Virginia truly deserved that award. I think her record for that year was twelve and a short two-month engagement, that she broke off after she got the diamond. And by the way, kept it, which added to her previous diamond collection from two other broken engagements. Yes, ole Virginia had a hobby: collecting diamonds; now she had an award for it. I told you she's clever.

Then came 1984, and we all, a few at a time, went on our excursion to flight school, and everyone came back with their versions and their stories about the things they did. Each of us who hadn't gone were more and more excited to go. We couldn't wait, and it seemed forever until our time would come.

Sooner or later, it did for each of us, and finally it was my turn. August 1984. I was on my way to San Antonio, Texas.

Four
Flight School

It would have been easier to take a plane from Sacramento to San Antonio. I was on my way to flight school. Airplanes and flight school seem synonymous, right? In retrospect I can easily see that I should have taken the hint. But I was going to be in Texas for six weeks and, understandably, I wanted my car while I was there. I also thought it might be fun to travel across the southlands by automobile. If I had flown, I would have missed the great travel-by-car adventure. Had I done that, I might have managed to live out my entire life without knowing what I know now. (Yet, in retrospect, I can honestly and unequivocally state that I would have preferred it that way!)

Everything was carefully planned. What I would need was carefully packed. When I left Sacramento, early that first day, I thought I had everything under control. I'd spent a lifetime in a profession where surprises and emergencies were dealt with in an efficient and confident manner. Maybe that's why the next twenty-four hours had such a topsy-turvy effect on me.

I'd spent a long, hot day traveling down the San Joaquin Valley. My destination was to be Edwards AFB for the first night. I could stay there at the officers' quarters, flirt a little with the test pilots, and feel safe. However, by the time I got to Edwards AFB it was too soon to stop, so I decided not to stop and headed on to Needles. That was a big town and I should be safe there. It can get mighty warm in the southern regions in August, and by the time I hit Needles, California, I was ready for a well-deserved rest. Needles was a somewhat dreary and dusty town sitting out in the middle of one of the most godforsaken deserts in the United States. At the same time, it was something of an oasis. If you didn't stop in Needles you had nowhere else to stop. I had to stop. I was tired and there was nothing for hours after Needles. However, later, I was sorry.

I must have spent half an hour driving around town before I pulled into what looked to be the nicest motel available, which in retrospect was not.

My car breathed a sigh of relief as it rolled to a stop between sun-faded strips of yellow paint. Outside, the air was heavy, stifling in its intensity, even though the sun had set hours before. I hadn't expected less. I'd been forced to close the vents on my dash the last hundred miles. Having nothing more than the desert heat to draw from, they blew only hot, fetid air, working more as heaters than coolers even at highway speeds.

The motel office was a beckoning splash of color and light, particularly the red neon "air conditioned" sign. I was tired and damp with perspiration, an icy bottle of champagne sat, still cold in the back seat of my car. At the last moment, I'd stopped at a mini-mart and bought it, a small celebration as well as welcome respite from heat, heat, and more heat. All I could think of at the time was to bless all-night grocers and this motel for being just a couple of blocks away from each other so my champagne would still be cool. I was in no state, nor did I have the right kind of experience (do any of us?) to judge the man who sat behind the counter of the place I intended to spend the night.

To me he was nothing more than a night clerk hyphen manager, one of that vast mass of people you come in regular contact with but never really think about. They do their job; you do yours. A day later, if you were asked, you wouldn't even be able to say with any certainty what color their hair was. Nonentities almost to a man. At some time—most of the time, one would argue—we are all members of this group. After awhile, we all take them for granted, not really seeing, hearing, or speaking to them. Then one will step out of the crowd, and everything changes.

I checked in as fast as I could, not even questioning the room I was given, even though it was up a flight of stairs and at the far end of the building, the last room in a long line of rooms. I was just so glad to be there, to rest, to cool off, to anticipate my future in Air Evac.

A small fly in the ointment occurred when I tried to turn on the air conditioner and the knob moved freely and the buttons pushed in then popped out but no fresh air was forthcoming. Yet, I still did nothing, opting instead to climb into the shower. It seemed easier than traversing the long walkway and steep stairs, suitcases in hand, to request a different room. And the water was wonderful. Cool, refreshing fingers of spray teasing my heated flesh, playing little melodies on my shoulders and breasts. I stayed under its rejuvenating torrent until the cold champagne beckoned, promising an even greater release from the heat of the night and the tension of the long drive.

I lay naked on the bed, slowly sipping away the smooth almond-flavored champagne until all of the tightness oozed from my limbs. Finally, not even caring about the broken air conditioner, I slipped into a light sleep.

A slash of light teased the edge of my consciousness.

I tried to ignore it, preferring instead to drift back into the gray area of twilight sleep I'd found so comforting just moments before. My mind wouldn't let me. Instinct dating back to primitive man will sometimes take over, even against our wishes. At that moment, it did, and my eyes opened, desperately trying to focus through the myopia of my astigmatism.

I saw little but the shadow of a man, haloed by the light that had awakened me, standing at the foot of my bed. My uncovered skin began to crawl, erupting in goose flesh and flashes of cold and hot. And another primitive reaction set in—pure, unadulterated fear. I was lying totally naked, my entire body exposed in a strange room in a strange town where no one even knew of my existence, and there was a strange man staring at me just inches from my feet. Simultaneously I needed to run, I needed to vomit, I needed to do anything to break the fear and shock-induced paralysis that gripped my throat and limbs.

It seemed to take forever to force a sound past the burning ball of bile that closed off my voice. "What are you doing here?" It was merely a rasp, but enough to break the emotional chains holding me in place.

"Get out of my room!" I sat bolt upright, snatching the wrinkled bedspread over my nudity. I threw a pointed hand toward the shaft of light.

"Get out!" My voice rose, not with the shrillness of fear, but with anger.

He wavered, his eyes hooded. Then abruptly, he was gone. He hadn't spoken a word.

For a long moment, I sat shaking on the bed, then, I jumped up and put on my glasses, not relishing taking the time necessary to replace my contact lenses. I didn't have much of my senses about me. I was still reeling from what had happened and the ugly possibilities of what it might have escalated to had he not left at my command. I wasn't even certain, as yet, how he had gotten into my room.

The click of a lock sounded through the cloud. My eyes fastened on the door that stood sentinel between my room and the one adjacent to it. A barely perceptible ribbon of light shone underneath, then magically disappeared. Even as my feet propelled me to the door, I wondered what I would do, what I could do. I knew I wanted to do something, I just couldn't form a tangible thought as to what. My hand curled around the doorknob. It was still warm. From the heat of the night? From the heat of his hand?

I shook and turned and rattled. I fought the desire to scream obscenities at the budge-proof handle. It was locked from the other side. I couldn't get through it. And one of my questions had been answered.

I stared at the door, thinking, *This must be a dream. This is really strange. Yes, I must be dreaming it all.* I wondered what to do. Not coming up with any good answers, I looked to tradition for solace and help. When one has trouble, the obvious response is to go to someone who is in charge. So I called the manager. No one answered.

For the dozenth time that night, I found myself confused, looking at the telephone as if it had a mind of its own. I suppose I was experiencing some sort of shock, because I didn't even question the reason the manager's phone would ring and ring with no answer. Instead, I slipped into slacks and a blouse, pulled on my stockings and shoes. Again I tried to reach the manager.

It was picked up on the second ring. "Yes?"

"Someone has been in my room." It sounded odd, hearing the words spoken out loud that way. I remember hoping he would believe my story and not think I was some kind of kook. "A man. He came in through a side door."

"Well," there was a long pause, "what do you want me to do about it?"

I stopped. I didn't have an answer. "I don't know." It was the best I could come up with, but I felt foolish saying it.

He was thinking. You could tell by the soft catches of breath slipping through the telephone receiver. "I'll make you a deal."

"Yes?"

"I'll give you your money back," he said carefully. "Then you can go to another motel. Would that be all right?"

"You've got it!" I was relieved beyond words. I don't know why I hadn't asked for that to begin with.

I was in a hurry to get out of there. I thought of very little else at that moment. My bags were packed in seconds. I didn't know where I was going to go or what I was going to do. The one idea I had, sleeping in my car, was quickly thrown out. I was still frightened. I was afraid that if I slept in my car someone would get me from it.

My thoughts continued to race. Could I find another motel? What if the man I'd seen was violent? What if he followed me—I wouldn't be safe even in a different motel. What would prevent him from doing the same thing again? *What if it was someone I knew, someone who, for whatever reason, had been following me and wanted to hurt me? What if there was no place I could go?*

I picked up the crumpled roadmap from the nightstand and sank onto the edge of the mattress. Kingman, Arizona, didn't appear too far down the road, but friends had warned me about the desert roads past Needles. I knew I was still too tired to drive. Add to that my emotional state, I didn't think it would be wise for me to continue on down the highway. Lake Havasu City looked closer, but traveling the snaky byway to it would be too demanding. I realized I'd already committed mistake number two. I'd driven too far in one day and wasn't really able to go on, considering the country I'd have to cross. I had no way of knowing whether, once out of Needles, there would be any motels open. It was already terribly late.

I knew exactly where I was, exactly where I needed to go, and yet I felt completely lost. I was completely panicky.

I stuffed the last of my things in my bag and went to the lobby for my refund. It was still swathed in light, the bright neon sign a fluorescent hue in the window, but now it had a garish quality. It was as if it said, "Come in, let me fool you. Let me take you." I shivered and stepped inside.

The manager lifted his head from the magazine he'd been browsing through, a slick patch of straight black hair slipping onto his forehead with the motion. Bland Mongolian eyes stared at me, almost daring me to speak. Snakes began to curl beneath my flesh, fastening their fangs on my muscles, crawling along my joints, wreaking havoc with my mind. He seemed to be enveloped in a fog, one that I had difficulty dispersing. On the counter before him lay bills and coins in the exact amount of my room bill. Reluctantly, my arm reached forward and my fingers closed over the money. I couldn't bear to have him touch me by allowing him to hand me the cash.

I said thank you, backed out the door, and hastily locked myself in the car. From my viewpoint behind the safely locked door, I could see the silhouette of the manager through the window of the office. He'd risen and stood watching from inside. The light walls behind him and outside reflections on the glass combined to create a halo effect. So I knew who had been in my room, violating my privacy, stealing my peace of mind. I got out of there as fast as I could, leaving nothing more than a thin strip of rubber in my wake.

I drove around town. I was tired, too tired to go on to Kingman or Havasu. I was scared. I'm the independent type, but right then I wanted more than anything someone to take care of me. God, I wanted someone to take care of me. I felt so incredibly vulnerable and alone. Then I saw a motel proclaiming "AAA Approved." It was like seeing an old friend. It's funny how a familiar word or sight can be so calming in stressful times. "AAA Approved" drew me like a magnet. The American Automobile Association is synonymous in this country with help. I pulled in and asked the lady in the night clerk's cage if she had any vacancies.

I grilled her, telling her my story, asking, "Is it a room without adjoining doors? Is it close to your office? Is there a double lock on the door?"

She gave me a key and assured me I'd be safe. Without even moving my car, I locked myself in the room. I stayed there, awake, watching television with all my clothes on until exhaustion overcame me and I fell into a fitful sleep. As soon as I awoke, I got myself together and left. I wanted out of Needles. I couldn't leave fast enough. I swore to myself that from then on, I wouldn't stay anywhere other than at an Air Force base.

Still, I couldn't exorcise the panic and fear. All day long I replayed the scenario and wondered. Even to this day, I don't have a solution, because with the panic that was inside me, I don't think I could have done anything. I only hope that the anger I felt that night had saved me. If he hadn't left when I told him to, it would have built into a burning rage. The panic immobilized me. The rage could have transcended that. It could have made the difference between life and death. I gave myself absolution with that thought. It was all I had. It had to be enough.

It kept me sane throughout the rest of the trip, which, fortunately, was fairly uneventful. That is to say, the events were pleasant rather than traumatic. I looked up an old friend, a helicopter pilot I'd once dated, in Albuquerque, and we had a great time touring Kirkland Air Force Base and dining at the officer's club. He was nice. We talked about old times, and it really helped me put the Needles trauma in the past.

There was only one more overnight stop before reaching San Antonio. It was Sheppard AFB, which was quiet and uneventful. The last leg of my trip had been hot, sultry, and extremely dull, but I'd made it—tired but eager, frightened but wise. They'd told me I was going to be going to survival school. However, I swear the drive from California to Texas (particularly through Texas in August) is survival school.

It wasn't much past noon, when I got to Brooks Air Force Base, so I went ahead and checked in. You always have to tell someone where you are and why, because they are accountable for you, and in this case were expecting you. I was thrilled to be assigned quarters, so I could finally unpack my things and classify a small area as home—and be safe, and sound. Excitement was beginning to build, and I eagerly went in search of a place to mingle and meet the people I would be studying with for the next six weeks. Sadly, as much as I longed for the primary contact, I met few people that day. But the next day was the first day of class and then the real adventure began!

The first day of flight school is organized insanity.

First, weigh-in. That was the first source of pain or pleasure. I was happy to know I easily fit in under the maximum weight a woman my height could be. If I hadn't they would have shipped me out. You're expected to fit the standard—or else. More than one sigh of relief escaped the lips of trainees on that day! At least you didn't have to worry about it from that point on. They only weighed you once. Which, as it turned out, was a godsend. There was some great food, and fantastic reasons to consume it in San Antonio, and a lot of us would have missed the second weigh-in if the Air Force had been cruel enough to stage one.

Classes began at 8:00 A.M. sharp. From then until 5:00 P.M., five days a week, we studied. And studied. And studied.

We covered the eight stresses of flight. Then learned even more about them until we could recite every nuance, every possible scenario by heart. At forty thousand feet, there is no room for error.

So we went over proper procedure to provide humidified air to patients who needed it; a dozen and more ways to deal with noise, nausea, fatigue, and G-force; how to deal with patients—and ourselves—when Boyle's law of gas resulted in painful (and sometimes deadly) build-ups of abdominal pressure; and why it's not particularly bright to drink and fly.

We set up in-flight incubators, checked oxygen lines, palpated blood pressure, changed dressings, dealt with changes in temperature, and learned what considerations must be made for anemia, tumors, colostomies, and more when carrying patients thousands of miles high above the clouds.

We learned how to nurse with limited use of stethoscopes, with the roar of props in our ears, with oxygen levels equivalent to working atop an eight-thousand-foot mountain peak and all the while keeping it all business, watch your words, keep those nails and hair short, always follow the code of ethics and, most importantly, always looking good while doing all this.

We discovered the differences between planes—like the C-141, C-130, and C-9; and found similarities—e.g., the doors were heavy, the ladders were swingy, the oxygen tanks were scary, the water gauges hard to find, and the first aid kit locations waiting to be memorized.

Yes, boys and girls, to be an Air Evac nurse, there's a *lot* to learn!

I'd expected classes to be incredibly exciting, but they can best be described as informative. Well, I guess that's what they should be, after all. Not that they were dull and boring, but it just seemed that they had a way of cutting into the time we spent goofing off. Hmm. Maybe I should rephrase that. Classes, which were titillating, educational experiences, were occasionally interspersed with moments of fun and comradeship with my fellow classmates. There. Doesn't that sound like a dedicated professional who is adequately immersed in her studies? Good. Now let's talk about the parties.

We all charged the officer's club en masse after the books were closed and our notes were transcribed. The first day was "get acquainted day." So we did. I immediately hit it off with a small group who had also just arrived. Terry was a beautiful Southern belle fresh in from North Carolina. Her voice could have melted ice caps in the Rockies. She always looked put-together and had the shiniest black crop of hair I'd ever seen. It framed her pale ivory face in graceful curves. She must have remembered me from check-in, because she pulled me to their table as I walked by.

"This is the nurse I was telling you about." Terry smiled. She had dimples. Somehow I could have guessed.

"Hi," I answered, then laughed. "Jim! I thought I saw you earlier. Wow. A long way from Mather, aren't you."

Terry didn't even skip a beat. She would make a great hostess, I thought. "You two know each other? I thought I heard you were from Tently Air Force Base, um, Lori, isn't it?"

"Yes. I'm in the 25th Air Evac, but Mather is far from unfamiliar territory for me. Jim and I are old friends. This is great."

"Sit down, Lori. What are you drinking?" I turned toward a distinctly masculine voice. Whoa. He was cute. He was also a flight surgeon. He stuck out his hand. Oops. A wedding band gleamed in the candlelight. "Call me Bishop."

"Okay, Bishop. Thanks." It's amazing how easily you can fall into friendships in the military. Perhaps it's because everyone is so far from home, we all make it a little easier to be friendly. Otherwise, it could be an extremely lonely profession. I took the nearest chair, my back to the door, just as a waitress appeared. "I'll have a Seven High."

"Tequila," a Southern-flavored tenor floated down the back of my neck.

"What?" I looked up into jet black eyes.

"This is Texas, ma'am. Tequila is almost a requirement. Besides, it gets you fuzzy on the edges so much faster, and being as this is the biggest-everything state, you're required to get even fuzzier." The corners of his full lips tipped into a mischievous grin. It was a total non sequitur, but laced with charm as it was, no one bothered to take it to task.

"Tequila it is, then," I told the waitress.

"Me, too." He smiled. She smiled, obviously falling under his spell, and turned to walk away.

"Make them doubles!" I called to her receding back. The crowd cheered, and I knew then and there that I'd found a new Group.

Bishop rocked back in his chair and eyed us from across the table. "I can see right now that the two of you are going to hit it off great. Lori, this is Tom, and don't let that Southern gentleman air fool you. He's a viper."

Tom feinted a left hook at his buddy. "Never."

The curly-topped brunette to Jim's right wrinkled her suntanned nose. "Flight surgeons. The scourge of Air Evac. I'm going to dance."

Terry volunteered Jim's services as a dance partner, not that he seemed to mind. Sandra had that outdoorswoman air that he'd always appreciated. I wasn't surprised to learn that she was from Florida. She looked sun-drenched and athletic.

The rest of us sat and sipped our tequila and talked. Tom seemed never to take his eyes off me, not even when Lynne, the other South Carolinian in our little group, sat down next to him. I was flattered. Lynne would have been quite a catch by any man's standards. Lynne wasn't the steal-your-man type, though. She turned out to be a good friend of mine. Tom turned into much more. Much, much more. Before the night was out, we had discovered an affection that was soon to grow.

Tom really was a nice Southern gentleman. He had the manners of a saint, a wonderful sense of humor, and an innate wit that set him far apart from most of the men I'd dated. Being with him was easy, he made me feel wonderful. Very, very special. Even though (or maybe because) he was twelve years younger than I, there were none of the difficult phases my previous relationships had gone through, no moments of uneasiness or tension from being unsure of our compatibility. That never happened with Tom.

We spent all our free time together. We did everything together, even at flight school. Because he was a doctor studying to become a flight surgeon, our classes were next door to each other. So we would meet during our breaks, meet for lunch, get together immediately after class, and go out for the evening. I confess I was dangerously close to falling in love. He seemed so gentle, so perfect for me.

One night we met after class, and he drove me into San Antonio to a little nightclub. Inside, the smoke-filled air lent a dreamlike quality to the shadows from candlelight tracing ghostly paths across the mirrored walls. It was a quiet, intimate club, with small booths lining the walls and tables for two scattered at discreet distances around the floor. Tom led me to a corner booth, the one furthest from the door, far away from all the rest.

Always the gentleman, he helped me behind the table, then sat next to me, our sides touching when he laid his arm across my back. His fingers laced themselves softly in the hair that rested in a loose pageboy on my shoulders. I felt . . . wonderful.

A waiter appeared out of nowhere with an icy bottle of very expensive champagne. Tom must have made arrangements before we arrived, which didn't really surprise me. He was always doing something romantic. We sat and talked. Tom and I could talk for hours. It was so special, the time I spent with him.

He'd seemed a bit edgy, though, and I couldn't quite put my finger on why. We'd known each other for about a week, and granted, there were a lot of things about each other we didn't know, but still, I was confused.

"Lori," Tom's hand traced against the curve of my neck. The familiar tingling began just below my navel. "I have something to tell you, but it's not easy."

I looked deep into his dark eyes. There was a sad, contemplative look in them. I expected the worst. "Just tell me."

He watched me quietly, seemingly looking for the right words.

"You're married, right?" I blurted out the words only to immediately wish I could take them back.

"Yes." It was a velvety whisper, barely audible. "Lori, I'm sorry. I wanted to tell you, but couldn't. You're important to me, more than you could ever know. But then I became afraid someone else might tell you, and that wouldn't have been fair, especially since my wife and I are separated."

I looked at him impassively. God, I wanted to believe him.

"That's okay, Tom." I worked on a smile. "You're separated from your wife because you're at flight school, and she's still in South Carolina? But she thinks everything's fine, right?" The smile failed miserably.

"No, no." His face clouded with uneasiness. "We really are separated. Ah, Lori, please believe me. I could have chosen not to tell you, but I didn't think it would be right. I care for you. Please."

I kept my gaze riveted to the tiny bubbles playing a languid game of chase in my champagne glass. I tried to ignore his warm hands caressing my shoulders and waist. And I believed him. What we had together was fabulous, far too special to ruin simply because he was separated from his wife, but not yet divorced. That would come sooner or later. At the moment, I dove deeply into our relationship, relishing it as intensely as I could. And it was one of the most exciting and romantic times I'd ever had. Up until then, I had never experienced such lightness. The weeks flew by with little heed to minutes and hours, only brief references to smiles, laughter, and kisses stolen at odd moments.

One night, just before he was due to graduate from flight school, we'd gone for a walk along the River Walk in San Antonio. It was a warm, languid summer night, and the fresh air caressed our faces. You could smell the river, but it was a clean, refreshing scent. Someone, somewhere had planted magnolias. Tom and I stopped to lean over the carved concrete railing, trying to peer deeply into the water.

And we talked. He wove a beautiful tale about me and him and the life we could lead if I would go back with him to South Carolina. Visions of green grass surrounded by a white board fence, graceful stallions running across the turf, and a very proper English cottage danced in my head. We talked about a lot of things that swayed my feelings toward him. And then one day he was gone.

Would I really be going to South Carolina? Just what had I meant to Tom, after all? I fell into a sea of depression. While Tom had been at Brooks, I'd spent so much time with him, my other friends had been put by the wayside. Now I found myself gravitating toward them. Understanding, they welcomed me back to the fold. But I still felt sad and alone. The depression began to deepen.

I had to find out for certain if my suspicions were correct. So I cornered Bishop. His answers were honest but heartbreaking. Yes, Tom was married. No, he wasn't likely to give up the security his wife offered. And yes, he had cared about me, but it was doubtful whether or not I could forgive him. It was over for me and the Southern gentleman. So much for dreams. So much for pastures and horses and idyllic nights before a big stone fireplace.

I only hope that Tom doesn't do this as a regular thing, that he doesn't keep a woman in every port and a string of romances strewn along his path. And I hope, though it may be from selfishness rather than graciousness, that some day his wife learns about him and takes away his security.

There was one saving grace that pulled me from the doldrums and made the rest of my stay at flight school fun, and that was nearby Fort Sam Houston. Fort Sam and the U.S. Modern Pentathlon horses reached out and pulled me like a magnet to a freighter.

An Army base, Fort Sam is the training ground for both the horses and the Army officers who race in the pentathlon. Those animals that had already served their time, so to speak, were put in the rental string. For four dollars I was able to take one out and ride the course. Immediately my spirits lifted.

If it's true that P.T. Barnum said, "There's a sucker born every minute," I must have hit upon four people hatched at just the right moment. My friends innocently agreed to go horseback riding with me.

Gee, maybe I should feel a little guilty. I mean, I said, "Want to go riding?"

And they said, "Sure. Sounds like fun. Does it matter that we don't know how to ride horses?"

So I said, "Mmm."

"We can handle it," they assured me.

"Could be some pretty feisty horses." I tried to give them an out.

"We can handle it."

"Could be some jumpers."

"We can handle it."

"No telling what kind of animal you might get."
"We can—"
"Okay, let's go." I smiled and led my little group of sheep to the slaughter.

Five

They Jump Horses, Don't They?

Way back when I was an LPN (Licensed Practical Nuse) I decided to go on to complete my education and become a registered nurse. I applied and was accepted by a very good nursing school. Immediately, I wrote to my father and asked him if he could send me enough money to cover tuition and other expenses. He sent me a check and I went out and bought a powerful red thoroughbred with the money.

Daddy forgave me.

I trained, then raced, Topah on the professional horse racing circuit. I've been an equestrienne almost all my life. When I was seven, my father took me on a pony ride. It was glorious. To this day I can still relive the magic of that first ride.

I was terribly excited as I climbed into what, at the time, seemed to be the cavernous depths of the front seat of the car. Today was the day, and I knew it! I just knew that I was going to be allowed to ride on the bright-eyed little horses that I had so far admired only from a (safe, according to my parents) distance. I was going to ride! Today! My body literally vibrated with anticipation.

The drive to the amusement park was interminably long. But as I have discovered again and again throughout life, some of the very best things are well worth waiting for, because before long, there I sat, blonde hair neatly tucked back with flashy satin ribbons, carefully pressed Peter Pan collar ever so slightly whispering around my neck. I like to think I sat that pony very smartly that first day. Oh, I was born to ride horses. It was my destiny to control the sleek, agile creatures who could run with the wind, grasping small snatches of sky with their hooves.

For years I begged, pleaded, promised, cajoled, and did anything and everything within my power to convince my parents that their fair-haired lass needed—deserved!—a horse.

No go. Instead, at the ripe old age of eleven, they shipped me off to camp. Camp Nightmare.

I wanted to go home. Oh, not that that particular camp wasn't nice enough. It was. And it wasn't that the counselors weren't good and kind. They were. But when I'd decided to become Lori, "equestrienne" and "world traveler," I didn't realize it meant leaving Mom and Dad at home and doing it alone. I got homesick and cried. And cried and cried and cried until some ingenious soul discovered that slapping me onto a saddle worked like turning off a faucet. On a horse, no tears. Zap. I suddenly became the only "jolly camper" who was allowed to ride daily rather than the prescribed thrice weekly. I was thrilled. They were thrilled. We all got along great, and by the time I left camp I wasn't homesick anymore.

By the time I hit my teens, I had it all figured out. Every chance I got, I would ride my bicycle or catch the bus across our little patch of Chicago to the horse stables. Methodically, I entered contests sponsored by a tobacco company to "Win a Thoroughbred." Sooner or later I would get my horse.

Guess again. Someone else won the thoroughbred. Fate was definitely dealing some gruesome blows. Somewhat resigned, I decided to become a nurse, not fully aware of what it would do for me, and to me, over the years—and also unaware that through it, I would get my thoroughbred and be able to travel.

So I found myself, some twenty-plus years later, at flight school, leading my merry band of buddies toward the pentathlon obstacle course at Fort Sam Houston. I had more than enough experience on horseback to know exactly what I was doing. I was a bad girl. A very, very bad girl.

We'd decided we were going to go out for a two-hour ride. Of course, I picked the biggest and most active horse out of the string for myself. A majestic midnight black thoroughbred, he was obviously the leader of the group. The rest of my friends mounted animals they chose based more on "look at his beautiful color" or "he looks friendly enough" than anything else.

Calmly, we steered into the forest. So far so good. Then I spotted a series of jumps that had been set up by the pentathlon trainers for use as a practice run, their equivalent of a little cross-country course.

Temptation. Oh, God, temptation! There I sat, surrounded by novices and nonriders. There before me was an equestrienne's heaven—the pentathlon training course. There beneath me was an animal that loved to jump, would indeed do so at the drop of a hat.

I said, a bit too eagerly, "You guys mind if I jump?"

Poor innocents. They said no.

I spurred my horse onto the course. Theirs, in sequence, followed. Like a line of perfect little soldiers, one by one each of them was carried on a joyride through space. Muscles bunching, the horses' legs extended and retracted in flawless symphony with the barriers along the jumping track and the rises and dips of the mogul run. To watch it was awesome. To experience it would take your breath away.

Boy, did I get in trouble afterward!

"Dead meat, Drew." Bishop glared with a beetlelike grimace. "You and the horse."

Sandra prodded her now excited animal down the path. "Cute, Lori. Really cute. What do you do for an encore? Send us flying off a cliff?"

Terry looked around nervously. Maybe she was looking for a cliff. Everyone else just squirmed in their saddles. Jumping a horse has an interesting effect on your fanny unless you know what you're doing.

I dropped my head and pretended I was sorry. They all squirmed and bitched the rest of the way around the track. Finally, we came full circle. There before me stood the start of the jumping course. I bit the inside of my lip. I was, I decided, going to behave myself.

Terry looked me straight in the eyes and formed each word in a smooth ladylike drawl. "Let's jump it."

My head whipped around toward the others, expecting mutiny. They all grabbed their reins tightly and set their jaws.

"Jump it!" They had the fever. It was great. Every time after that when we rode, they begged to jump. Again and again they wanted to go back and do the mogul run. And they did. Those novice horseback riders became experienced very very quickly. What a pack of wolves my flock of lambs had become!

I wondered at the time, and still do, how I ever managed to keep up with them. They were all thirty-one, thirty-two, and I was thirty-nine. They were wild and crazy and had an innate ability to get me into trouble way over my head. Every night they wanted to go out to dinner or have a party. Somehow I kept up with them. Don't know how, but I did. Even when they went to the Irish Rose, a popular local sing-along bar.

Oh, brother, what a night. At one point I found myself on the piano, singing. Later, I thought nothing of carrying on a loud and vigorous peanut fight between bouts of consuming huge doses of Mexican food. One of my favorite photographs is the one of us hanging three at a time from a restaurant sign. Wild and crazy, it was a great time had by all.

So, in deference to those noble friends who so gallantly followed on horseback over hill and dale—not to mention air—I'll cut this chapter of our lives very short. By the time we'd come out of our trees, it was time for survival training. (Besides, their mothers might be listening.)

Six

Survival of the What?

Survival training. Or how to be made a fool of by a sixteen-inch armadillo in three easy steps. Are we having fun yet, guys?

There were about sixty of us due to be dumped in the desert for survival training. The powers that be divided that number into five groups. Oh, goody. Now I had the problem of being stuck in the wilderness with a group of know-it-all nurses that I hadn't even liked in the classroom. I didn't really think that I'd develop a deeper affection for them when we were all fighting for our lives in the middle of a Texas desert. And it was just my luck that my friends were all put together in a group and I got sloughed off with the worst of the worst. The Perfect Squad we called them.

I don't know what it is about some people that makes them so impossible when they're in a position of power or responsibility. But this particular bunch of groupies had damn near every bad quality I could think of. They spent all their time trying to show they were a little smarter than the rest of us. Nothing pleased them more than one-upping one of their peers or coming down on someone they considered an underling. Gag. Not one of the Perfect Squad would I have considered a friend, or even friendly, as far as that goes.

There were only two people in my band of happy

campers who were worth spending any time with. Jason was an extremely kind-hearted comic who, I swear, would have found a humorous side to major surgery. Lee tried, but couldn't do much of anything without stopping and starting, stopping and starting. He wasn't stupid. He was just so anxious to please, he would sometimes get in his own way. Both of them were male med-techs. Both of them were very young. And both of them, for obvious reasons, were considered by the Perfect Squad to be below them. I was also an outcast—it was my sense of humor, I guess.

So we went off to be outcasts together. Everyone else just continued to be self-absorbed with their serious thoughts and arrogant games. Bullshit, pure and simple. I'm sure some day they'll all be president.

Jason, Lee, and I shared a tent and did our best to stay out of everyone else's hair. (In the long run, it was easier than listening to and putting up with their garbage.) We'd fallen in together from the very first when a big blue Air Force bus had pulled up to load everyone, lock, stock, barrel, and C-rations, for the trip to no-man's-land. While the Perfect Squad was mentally calculating loading patterns for efficient transfer of survival equipment, we were taking pictures with Kodaks and sifting through C-rations.

We set up camp the first day. Lee and I got the tent together with a minimum of thumbs, then went over to help Jason and the others set up the mess tent. The next order of business was to catch dinner.

Wait a minute . . . *catch* dinner? I'm afraid that's not too easily done. Have you ever chased an armadillo? Or a snake? Or even a rabbit?

Conscientiously, we set our traps. Patiently, we waited. Eventually, we dined on dried-up cornflakes from our C-rations. At least I was warm all night. Sharing a tent with two guys provided me with two warm bodies to generate heat. All completely aboveboard, I guarantee. There were, after all, a whole group of trainees within sound distance.

The first night wasn't so bad. We crawled into our tents and collapsed. Sleep was quick to come but hard to keep. Sleep, awake, sleep, awake. First the Air Force spoils you with luxury rooms, then throws you out onto a snake-infested, twig- and rock-strewn patch of dust and nettles. I spent half the night marveling that I'd actually looked forward to this.

The next day, we tried once again to capture a little fresh meat. Our traps yielded nothing, so we set off on a hunt. I was walking on point, when one of the little armor-clad creatures scurried across the ravine ahead of me.

Dinner!

"Armadillo! Armadillo!" I screamed. (Okay, it sounds stupid, but you try screaming it. Not too easy, huh?)

We took off like maniacs. One thing is for certain, armadillos only look slow. They run like wildfire. We spent a half-hour chasing that little devil and probably expended twice the calories we would have consumed had we actually ended up eating him. At one point, we had him cornered in a low-lying patch of sagebrush, but—and I don't know how—he managed to sneak out. In the end, all we had were scratched hands, sore feet, and dirty faces.

One of the instructors took pity on us, though, and to compensate for the gallant effort we'd put out, gave us one they'd caught. Come to think of it, that particular instructor's group had a whole mess of snakes, rabbits, and armadillos. I wondered how they did it. Maybe they were lucky enough to have all the stupid animals in that stretch of desert snooping around their traps. Or maybe they were just good at trapping. Probably both.

Lucky for me I didn't have a queasy stomach. Quite a few people didn't relish eating armadillo stew. Once or twice I caught someone looking a bit green around the gills. I thought it was great though. We had armadillo stew, soup, and even roast. It beat emaciated cornflakes any day. Our traps never did offer up a deer or fowl. And nary a rabbit for the outcasts. I tried to tell myself that I preferred not to munch down on the Easter bunny anyway. It didn't work. By the end of the third day, there weren't many in our merry band who wouldn't have charged Rudolph the red-nosed reindeer with an eye toward charcoal-broiled steak.

By then we'd marched across miles of desert, putting up with itchy, dry throats, searching out water, eating little, and sleeping less. We were tired, smelly, and we looked awful. We were also so bad-tempered, no one was speaking to anyone else. Most of the women were fighting with each other, and eventually, people were kind of left by themselves.

The exception was the outcasts. Lee, Jason, and I had gone in with the point of view that we would make the best of what was almost guaranteed to be a bad situation. And we'd maintained a good sense of humor throughout. On the last night, we fell into the tent and began our good-night ritual.

I peeked into my sleeping bag. No snakes, no spiders. Exhausted, I squirmed in.

"Good night, Jason," I whispered.

"Good night, Lori," Jason replied.

"Good night, Lee," I said, louder this time.

"Good night, Lori," Lee pulled his cap over his ears.

"Good night, Lee," Jason's voice broke the silence of the night.

"Good night, Jason," Lee croaked, starting to warm

to the plot underway.

"Good night, John Boy," we squealed in unison.

"Shut up, you idiots!" a baritone laden with irritation retorted from another tent.

"God, what a pain in the ass," another voice mumbled from the other side of the campground.

"If they don't stop doing that, I'll kill them." The speaker was feminine, but not particularly sweet. "I swear to God I'll kill them."

"I'll loan you a gun," the baritone promised.

The three of us burst into giggles and laughed ourselves to sleep.

The next morning, we packed up and trudged to a common meeting ground, where we joined the rest of the groups. Once again the sixty of us were divided into teams. The object of this, our last exercise, was to set up a helicopter landing pad. The officer in charge told us to get it done fast and get it done right. A helicopter was actually going to be coming in within half an hour.

One team gathered supplies and marked the ground with a large X. One team set up the signaling, another the alarm. A fourth was in charge of communications. None of us had ever done anything like this before. Worse, directions from the instructors were brief and hurried.

Tired as we were, we rushed through the preparations and had the landing pad ready. A helicopter was going to come and take us back to the base! We sat and waited. And waited. After an hour, we began to wonder where our beloved helicopter was, how were we going to get back to the base.

Someone got brave and asked. Considering the fact that this particular officer had actually inflated raw armadillo lungs to show their use as a flotation device, it was a true act of bravery.

"There isn't going to be a helicopter," he said, and I swear there was a cruel gleam in his eye, "just training practice."

Fortunately the buses arrived at that moment, the instructor saved from dismemberment at the hands of sixty half-crazed nurses and med-techs. It could have been nasty. We all knew a lot about anatomy, and it would have been painful.

It would have been nice to fall head-first into a bath when we got back, but that would have been too easy. Instead, we all sat in a hot warehouse for a two-hour debriefing. Not too neat, considering we'd all been in the wilderness for days. Smelly, tired, hungry, the last thing we needed was to be told in detail how we'd spent the last few days. We knew how we had. Believe me, the memory would be vivid for quite some time, and analysis of the event was redundant as far as we were concerned. Therefore, it was a very long two hours.

But time clicks on, and eventually they turned us loose to attack candy-bar machines, remove six inches of grime under a blessedly civilized shower, and fall on a comfy bed for twelve straight hours of sleep. I have to brag, though, because when all my young buddies declared it official celebration time and headed to a seafood restaurant, I trudged along. Quite a few glasses of wine and plates of fish later, I realized I was having a great time. Being with all those young guys made me realize something else, too. Commercial clichés aside, I was not getting older, I was getting better!

The next day was graduation day.

The air around Brooks vibrated with excitement. We'd all come so far and done so much just to reach that special moment when they pin those wings on our sharply creased blue jackets. For most of us, years and years of education had preceded our military enlistment. Some, like me, had put in as many as six to eight years of school and many, many more years beyond that in hospital and clinic work. Endless forms, examinations, and waiting had to be waded through before we'd been officially sworn in to the Air Force. We'd come from air bases all over the country and spent months in orientation and preliminary training. But our time had finally come. The last six weeks of training and survival school had been overcome.

There was a moment as I put on my dress blues when I stopped and wondered, *Is this real? Is all of this really happening to me?* It seemed so incredible. Reminiscing to when I'd learned I could never be a stewardess and, consequently, would probably never fly, I felt unreal, unsure. Had I made it after all? Had I transcended the difficulty with my kidneys, the one that had grounded me so effectively all those years before? Had I really passed all the tests? Filled out all the forms? Been capable enough in my nursing? Or was I going to wake up and find it had all been a dream?

I ran a hand up my leg, straightening the nylons I'd put on seconds before. My scratched fingers moved roughly over the tan fabric. I stopped and turned my palms to my face. A long gash—not deep, just a surface mark, really—etched its way from the base of my index finger to my thumb. "Sagebrush bites," Jason had dubbed them. I'd gotten it diving for armadillo in a bleak Texas desert. I raised my eyes to the mirror, and a smartly clad blonde looked back at me. The dark blue uniform, pale shirt, perfectly folded tie framed her face. Was that fear in her eyes? A little apprehension maybe? No, no, I smiled at my reflection. It was exultation. Ignoring the cut on my hand, I smoothed the last stray hairs into place and closed the door behind me.

An hour later, Colonel Megan West stood before me, showing me my future.

"Ladies and gentlemen," her voice was clear and strong and proud, "the Pentagon has sent me here to talk to you about the lives you will be living as Air Force flight nurses and medical technicians." Carefully she folded her hands on the podium, pushing aside the stack of cards before her. Her eyes scanned us all one by one, and she took a deep breath. "But I would be here even if they hadn't sent me. You see," she said, "you are the best of the best. You are the people who are going to be the guardians of life. There will be times when the only thing that stands between a soldier living . . . and dying . . . is your skill and your faith. It won't always be easy, although your training is going to always serve you in good stead. It won't always be fun. You will cry, and die, a little with each battle lost. Yet, it is your province to forever strive for perfection. If anyone can achieve it, you will. This is true or you wouldn't have made it this far.

"I won't try to fool you," she said, and her chin lifted an almost imperceptible inch higher, "this is one of the toughest jobs anyone can take on. Twenty years ago, I found myself a lifeline for hundreds of wounded soldiers in Vietnam. And I was afraid. But they needed me, just as your patients will need you. When bullets were flying and bombs were exploding, . . . when young men, too young to understand, turned to me and said, 'Help me,'" Colonel West paused, swallowed deeply, "I helped. And so shall you. Because you are committed to excellence. Because you are committed to a standard far higher than that of ordinary man. Because you are Air Evac. And that makes you very, very special."

She raised her hand to the wings pinned on her chest. "Very special indeed. Occasionally, it may seem that you need wings on your back—angel wings—as well as the ones we'll be putting on your chest today. But no matter what nature or man puts before you, no matter what obstacles you may need to cross, your nobility will overcome them. It's part of the heritage that is Air Evac. And when all is said and done, look back and be proud. It's a right you will have earned."

She stepped away from the podium and stretched her arm toward the table at her side, the one that held the honors soon to be passed on to us.

"It is with great pleasure and deep honor that I introduce the newest members of our small but special branch of the Air Force." In her hand I saw them, my wings. I took a deep breath and stood as I'd done in our rehearsal exercises.

"Captain Lori Drew," Megan West looked me straight in the eyes; in that second she was both a military colonel and a woman, "Congratulations. You are now an Air Evac nurse."

She pinned the large silvery wings over my heart and took my hand in hers. I'd made it.

And it was all worth it. All the time, all the study, everything. I had never been prouder in my life.

Later that afternoon, I got into my car and began the drive back to California. As I pulled onto Interstate 10, I felt a small pang of sadness. I was leaving a lot of good friends, a lot of good times, and, yes, even a little bit of Texas behind.

Seven
Getting Qualified

Sitting sentinel on acre upon acre of blacktop, the huge green frame of a C-141 signaled its intentions. "Give me the new ones," it seemed to grunt, "I'll give them a hell of a ride."

I knew it was talking to me. I was fresh back from flight school, and the active duty nurse back at Tently was eager to get me qualified. In essence, I had graduated from training, and now I had to prove—that is, be tested under actual conditions—that I knew all the right stuff and could carry out my job. It takes at least four, but no more than six flights to get qualified. The active duty nurse wasn't the only one who wanted me to fly. I was eager, too.

I was buddied up with an instructor who would show me the little ins and outs I hadn't learned at flight school. I was assigned as flight nurse, and the instructor was there to show me how to set up my station on the aircraft and how to do paperwork, direct med-techs, and service patients. I was scared but excited and really wanted to do well. I found out that flight school really didn't prepare one for the pressures of actual flight.

Sometimes you had to wait in line to get a flight, but this time they needed nurses. There's a good reason I was able to get on that flight. It was headed for Alaska. No one except a few of us gung-ho types were willing to take off to Alaska in October. And so it began, my first flying experience. Not quite what I'd expected at that first Christmas party . . .

Out of bed at 3:00 A.M. and off to the base. Report in at 4:00 A.M. and get briefed by the medical crew coordinator, who is the nurse from the hospital to tell you about each patient, including what's wrong with them and what kind of special treatments and medications they'd be needing.

Drink a lot of coffee and eat a few donuts while being briefed; get instructions from the medical crew director (MCD) in charge regarding preparation of the plane; obtain, document, and store equipment and medications; examine configuration chart and see that everyone is placed where they should be (children on bulkhead, parents to their side, psych patients on bottom stanchions, critical care at waist level, and so on); have ground crew check configuration at aircraft; go over checklist for cardiac arrest, emergency procedures, ditching, crashing, meals; and the big one, who's in charge here?

Whoa! Are we done yet?

Then, call the crew bus and send an ambulance and fire truck to the flight line; take a bus to the plane; meet the pilot and memorize the tail number of the aircraft; have the MCD talk to the crew chief to see if it's time to board; board plane and set up oxygen masks; have the MCD survey the plane by checking emergency oxygen, first-aid kits, fire extinguisher, hatchets, ropes, rubber rafts.

There were fifteen of us on this training mission, which meant that five of us were going to fly in crew positions, the rest assigned various maladies to become "instant patients" for us to practice on. Crew members play good patients because they are trained and aware of the symptoms of the diseases they will be simulating. At the FCC's (Flight Crew Coordinator's) command, they enact medical emergencies during the flight so the crew's response and care could be effectively evaluated. No small task, considering the four trunks of equipment, litters, and luggage that are configured in the back of the plane and are usually in the way. If you have a cardiac arrest you have to pull the patient onto the floor of the aircraft and pump away. (It happened and it was tight!)

So we take a deep breath before the officer of the day walkie-talkies a go-ahead to bring the patients to the flight line; the flight nurse escorts her ambulatory patients to their assigned seats; every available arm helps to load the litters, strap them in, check the patients' IVs, vital signs, dressings, and equipment. Then comes a briefing over the loudspeaker regarding safety, similar to the ones you'd hear aboard a commercial flight—umm . . . this is a life jacket, inflate it this way . . . this is oxygen, use it so . . . seat belts—and more.

And takeoff. Maybe. Providing nothing has gone wrong, and it had better not. In the USAF, if the plane is due to take off at 8:00 A.M., you can bet that it'll be taxiing down the runway at 7:45. If a patient needs your constant care, they'd strap you to his stanchion and you'd be standing there, strapped in, doing your job while the plane takes off—all of the way to 42,000 feet.

And those are the necessary preparations just to get airborne. Obviously Air Evac is not all fun and games, although there is plenty of that, too. It's also good, honest, hard work, the kind of work that, when done right, makes a difference. And it really hits home the first time you try to do ten things at once in a rumbling airplane.

During all this, Linda, the instructor who was training me, kept up an ongoing monologue of rules of thumb and hints to help ease the pressure and make it all a bit easier. Each instructor has their own way of teaching, and I was really glad I had Linda. Of course, I was green and didn't know how to do any of this stuff. I confess to being a little scared, too. But I was all eyes and ears and willing to learn anything I could. Boy, did I! I spent a lot of years garbed in a nurse's uniform, and I must say that with every moment I practiced my craft—not only in Air Evac, but in all the other places I worked, as well—there was something new and wonderful to learn. And the more I learned, the more I practiced, and the longer I worked, the better it got.

Working in synchronization, like a fine Swiss watch, generates a feeling unlike any other. It's special. I wish that everyone at some time in their life could find themselves in a situation where the job is going smoothly and everything is falling into place. In an odd way it reminds me of those marathon domino displays. Every domino that falls does so in a way that makes the slide continue. You keep expecting one of those little black chips to slip a little too far to one side, but it doesn't, and the show just continues on its well-oiled way. It's spectacular. Just like good nursing.

I learned a lot on that first Alaska mission. There was so much new and helpful knowledge to digest. I learned to do a lot of things. I learned a few things not to do, too.

Mama Cherise from orientation was the medical crew director on that flight. An interesting thing happened when the title MCD was slapped on Cherise's back. She turned from Mama into a drill sergeant. In her defense, I can say that being medical crew director is a hard job with a lot of built-in pressures. And it's not as if she bound any of us with surgical tape and dropped us out the door as we were landing or taking off. It was more a matter of pulling rank, I guess. The MCD had a tremendous amount of responsibility riding on her shoulders. It was serious business, but some nurses took it too seriously.

On any given flight, there's one person who knows that plane inside and out, upside down, right side up, and all the points in between. He's an enlisted man, and they call him the loadmaster. There is to some extent amongst some military personnel an innate snobbery attached to whether one is enlisted or commissioned. Generally, someone who is enlisted came into the service and learned a trade. He was, in essence, taught by the government to do a job for the government. If, however, he is commissioned, he signed into the service already skilled in a trade the government found valuable or he had an advanced education. Uncle Sam said, "Hey, look at you. You're bringing brains to the USAF, USMC, whatever, and so we'll make you an officer." While a lot of us figure a skill is a skill is a skill, there are those who think they're a little better than everyone else if they didn't acquire theirs dressed in olive drab.

This isn't strictly a military problem. It surfaces in almost every facet of the working world, and in some social circles as well. (You mean you aren't an alumnus of Hahvahd? How droll.) But give a person a little responsibility and add to that some power and rank. Zap. Instant drill sergeant.

I was disappointed in Cherise's attitude. I'd held her in high regard, but when I saw her bossing people around and forcing herself into a position of power, I was a bit put off. I knew that it wasn't the way I wanted to be when I made MCD. I don't think you have to dictate to your people when you want things done.

Mama Cherise probably didn't realize that. In the final analysis, the pilot and the loadmaster are the ones in charge. Some nurses just didn't seem able to accept that.

Cherise was one of them. But I learned a lot from watching her and the rest of the crews' reactions to her. And I didn't let it get to me. I figured that I was there to learn, and any kind of direction, kind or not, that someone gave me was to be valued. In the end, I drew on my years as an intensive care nurse and followed my instincts to look at the lighter side of things. It helped.

This was, though, to be an indication of things to come. As I got into it, one of the most difficult facets of Air Evac was problems with in-crew tensions. It was only to be expected, I suppose, with so many people doing such a stressful job under difficult circumstances. But I never understood where everyone was hiding their sense of humor. We had a great time on the ground, but in the air . . . sometimes it was duck and hide.

It wasn't so bad, though. Alaska was breathtaking, even in the dark, and I got some extremely important flight nurse training in. I got a lot of studying done, and I had a wonderful time laughing and talking with all the men I met who were also stopping over in Alaska while I was there. The trip back to California was strained but basically uneventful, and I managed pretty well even when I was given hypothetical emergencies to handle them.

By the time I got back, I felt I was ready to go on a training flight that would count toward getting me qualified as medical crew director. There was more pressure being MCD than being the flight nurse, consequently, if you had qualified as an MCD, you were automatically qualified as a flight nurse. I was eager to get through this important training period, so I took a training flight to Japan and back.

There were twenty-five of us on that mission, most of us students. And then there was Virginia Starr. Gee, I was real lucky! I had Virginia Starr along as an instructor. Fortunately, my immediate instructor was someone else. Virginia was in charge of watching Grandma Betty, who was trying to pass her flight instructor certification. Not that Virginia didn't manage to annoy even those on her periphery. I mean, we were locked in an airplane flying over miles and miles and miles of ocean with her all the way to Guam, the Philippines, and Japan and back. We're talking *days* here. I was sweating before we even took off.

We had to put in special effort on this flight, too, because my friend Dixie and I were both being trained as medical crew director. That meant we had to set up two stations on the C-141, which we'd nicknamed the lizard. Okay, we could have handled that. I had a wonderful instructor, Della, who was just a dream, and Grandma Betty was in charge of Dixie's training. Virginia was in charge of everything because she was a flight examiner and had to evaluate all training.

So there we were, twenty-five people in a huge green airplane, the rumble of the jet engines making it difficult to hear much of anything, not to mention reams and reams of paperwork, plus patient care. And we had to spend five days and cross six time zones with a woman who had nothing better to do than to claw us all in the back. Neat trip. However, even though things got a little tight now and then and tempers tended to flare, I worked hard at trying to maintain my sense of humor. If ever there was a cause I'd jump on the bandwagon for, it was keeping your good humor throughout, no matter what. This was one of those times when it wasn't easy.

But we survived—some of us actually were unscathed—and I must say that the ground time on that voyage was pure enchantment. Hawaii, Guam—so much beauty.

Della was incredibly understanding when she discovered how excited I was about seeing those wonderful new places. Instead of loading me up with heavy study time, she told me what I needed to know and let me loose to explore. And I did, we all did. Hawaii beckoned.

A pilot from headquarters invited us all to a party in his room. Afterwards, we went jogging. Let me tell you, jogging on Oahu, Hawaii, transcends exercise. It's no wonder there are so many healthy-looking people wandering that island.

Most of the beaches are a narrow band of pale, pale champagne. And if you watch closely, there are tiny crabs not much larger than your thumb that scamper across the sand just as you approach. You can hear the wild doves cooing in the trees. The palm fronds seem to whisper exotic songs in the warm, steady breeze that constantly caresses your skin, not unlike a gentle lover. The ocean itself has a jewellike quality, as if it were a giant aquamarine, flashing this way and that, mellifluously reflecting the sun's rays. It's a sensory experience that can lift you up into a calm and meditative state. All that's asked is to just allow yourself to be moved.

It was a much appreciated respite before we boarded the C-141 for the next leg of the trip, Guam. It gets confusing flying half the way around the world. Although it was only an eight-hour flight to the base on Guam, halfway there, we crossed the International Date Line. Simply put, we left early Sunday morning and arrived at about three o'clock Monday afternoon. Although we'd been in the air for only eight hours, a good twenty-eight hours showed on the clock.

As soon as we unloaded and placed our medications under safe lock and key, we headed for food. Billeting had placed us in an off-base hotel on the beach, which was nice. The food in the restaurant was nice. The company I was with was nice. Everything was nice, except for my eyes, which insisted on drooping closed. My body didn't know that I was enjoying good food and good conversation on a tropical island at five in the afternoon. It thought I was in Sacramento, California, ready to doze off at one o'clock in the middle of the night.

I fell asleep in my scallops. One of our med-techs, Gary, extricated me. Lucky. If he hadn't, my epitaph would have read, "Drowned in clarified butter her heart flew, but her head sagged." Grim. Buddies that they were, they carted me off to my quarters and tucked me away. Thanks, friends.

Slowly my eyes opened, and small traces of sunlight filtered into my drowsy brain. As I finally regained consciousness, I went into a panic. I didn't know for sure what time or even what day it was. I'd gone through so many time changes and worked such odd hours, I'd completely lost track of the clock. I was scared to death that I'd overslept and botched the whole mission. Since I was acting medical crew director, I had to be in charge of the flight and everybody on it.

The mathematics involved in calculating time changes on this kind of a mission are monstrous, especially to a frightened, dazed mind. It seemed as if I never would, but eventually I did get a grip on it and realized that I hadn't overslept, but had actually underslept. I was up three hours early. It was only 3:00 A.M. Guam time. I resisted the temptation to check my pulse, even though I was sure it was going at aerobic speed without the benefit of exercise, and went for a walk along the beach.

The astonishing thing was that it really was light at three in the morning. Halfway between the Equator and the Tropic of Cancer, the Mariana Islands are even more tropical than Hawaii. And Guam could easily be the most beautiful of them.

I had never seen anything quite as overwhelming as Guam in the wee hours of the morning. I walked along the beach, making small dips in the crystalline silver sand, listening for the foamy opaline breakers as they rushed to greet the shore. Wide bands of leaf green, the expressive fingers of the palms, reached for me as I passed, promising to deliver ticklish delights if I ventured very close. On my one side, sapphire waves rose and crested in a timeless dance with the moon; on my other, emerald grass peeked in tiny wisps from beneath exotic honey-colored flowers. It was entrancing. Guam wove a hypnotic spell, pulling into its web any who ventured onto its surface.

Two of the med-techs had also gotten up early and saw me wandering the beach and came out to join me. Were they immune to the beauty there? Or did they only see it for a different purpose? They challenged me to a race, and off we went down the length of snowy sand. I don't know who won. I think we all did. As we ran, I could imagine, if only for a moment, what it must have been like all those centuries ago—before World War II and the bunkers and bullets and battles; before civilization stamped its discordance on the land; before missionaries with their new laws and strange customs came—back to when native girls and boys lived peacefully and played blithely in nature's own empire. It must have been good. It must have been very, very good.

That's the Guam that I took away with me when we boarded the plane for the Philippines that morning. That's the one I think I'll keep forever. I don't really want another.

I'd signed up to travel, though, so Uncle Sam plucked

me from a tropical paradise and sent me to the Philippines. The Philippines used to be paradise, too, I hear, until mankind squished its face. It still has some nice areas, and a lot of the people are friendly. But it was so frenetic in Manila, and Clark Air Force Base was surrounded by so much insanity, it was hard for me to feel too thrilled about being there. It was quite different from Sacramento, that's for sure.

The Philippines was the first place we'd been that wasn't under U.S. control. Immediately upon our arrival, a group of Filipino officials brought police dogs on board to search for illegal drugs and spray the plane before we went through customs. We carry real medications, even on training flights, some of them are controlled narcotics and they need to be locked up at the base dispensary. Because there was a huge overseas exercise going on at Clark when we got there, space for such things, as storing medications, was very hard to come by. We'd already tried ordinary channels to no avail. And that's when Virginia grimaced, and we knew terrible things were about to transpire.

"Philip," she whimpered to one of the airmen who'd come in with us, "isn't there anything that can be done? Isn't there anywhere we can lock up these medications? I'm so tired I can barely stand." She stared at him seductively.

Phil shrugged his massive shoulders. He'd spent two years in Vietnam and another two running the Manila Playboy Club. There seemed to be very little that could faze him. Not even Virginia Starr. He just walked away and dropped his flight bag in the hall so he could use the phone.

Virginia pursed her lips into a tight line and narrowed

her eyes. Surprisingly, she didn't go after him. Instead, she accosted a thirtyish master sergeant who'd been watching it all from a vantage point behind his desk. Virginia turned on the charm.

"Excuse me, Sergeant, but would you mind if I sit down?" She sounded as if she was going to expire at any second.

"No, make yourself at home." The sergeant cleared his throat and went back to writing neat little numbers on the forms before him.

Virginia smiled. Make yourself at home. We all knew that Sergeant Mallory was a goner. Ignoring the ugly chrome and Naugahyde chair several feet away, Virginia positioned herself provocatively on the edge of his desk, not more than five inches from his bare forearm. Now, there's an interesting thing about flight suits. They look good on Tom Cruise. But they look great on a slim-hipped, full-busted woman. Virginia made pretty good show of fanning her cleavage with the sheafs of documentation we'd been carrying around in our search for lockup space. It was both disgusting and fascinating. I found myself wondering, *Will this guy fall for that? It's so obvious!*

"Our friend is renting a bus for us all." She leaned back and rested on her open palms. "We're all going to the Playboy Club. You know, in Manila. Have you ever been there?"

The sergeant looked up from his task. "No, can't say as I have."

"I hear it's nice."

"So I'm told."

"You can come along with us if you'd like." There it was. The Virginia Starr kill-them-in-their-tracks smile.

"Thanks," the sergeant said before dropping his head back to his papers, "but I have to work."

"Oh, we'll be there for a long time. Maybe you can drop by afterward?"

"No, sorry." The sergeant flipped a couple of pages into a file folder.

Had it happened? Had Virginia Starr met her match in this rather mousey little man with the metal rimmed glasses? We waited anxiously. Virginia watched the sergeant pensively.

"You've been in almost twenty years I'll bet. Right, Sergeant Mallory?" she said tiredly.

"Twenty years in another nine months, ma'am." He barely lifted his eyes from the desk.

Good guess, Virginia, I thought, *but what is this leading to?*

"My father was a thirty-year man himself." Virginia stood up, stretched her back, and loosened the Velcro tabs cinching the fabric around her waist, instantly hiding a good portion of her curves. She paused a second and lowered the boom. "Enlisted."

She was good. I had to give her that. Of course, I doubted that she even had a father. More than likely some evil witch had brewed her from toad tongues and bat hair in some slimy cauldron deep within the Black Forest. Even if someone would admit to parenting her, it was unlikely he'd spent thirty years in the Air Force. But ten minutes later the sergeant had found a safe place for us to store our medications and we were on the bus headed for Manila. What sex hadn't acquired, loyalty had. Or maybe, and this is my favorite theory, the sergeant did it just to get her out of there so he could finish his paperwork. Whatever, it was one of the few times I was actually happy to have the illustrious Ms. Starr along.

True to his word, Phil had chartered a bus for the ride to the Playboy Club, and we all anxiously awaited a night on the town. The ride into Manila was enough excitement; it can only be likened to something they'd build at Magic Mountain Amusement Park to scare the daylights out of you. In the PI, people drive like crazies, cutting in and out, jamming on brakes, swerving and swarming, all of the while alternating between outrageous speeds and a turtle-like crawl in their tattered and wildly decorated rigs. Phil assured us that it was always like that, that we hadn't gotten involved in some bizarre road race.

By seven o'clock, about fifteen of us were being escorted to fabulously prepared tables in the Playboy Club. All the employees put out a special effort to treat us like royalty. Phil was something of a celebrity there, and all stops were pulled for this visit. They even put on a special show for us.

We had to get back to the base by midnight, but until then we had a great time. All the tables were set with white linen, crystal goblets, and long white tapers in silver candlesticks. Bunnies clad in maroon velvet, white tux collars, and black bow ties waited on us hand and foot. It was nice to sit there with friends, be treated like kings and queens. It was definitely different than some of the back-roads bars I'd stopped off in during my drive through Texas!

All good things come to an end, though, so eventually we trudged off to the bus and took the kamikaze route back to Clark. The next morning we had to fly the rest of the way to Japan.

We were lucky; a delay prolonged our layover in Japan from just a few hours to two days, which meant we had plenty of time to *shop!* Flashes of Mary's stories of shopping suddenly ran through my head.

The beauty of Air Evac is that good old Uncle Sam gives you a paycheck for being a nurse. Then he says, "But of course you'll need something extra because you're so sweet to go to all these strange places for me. Here's a per diem to cover additional expenses." Thanks, Sam! Our per diems made great trinket money, especially since the government paid for our hotel expenses.

Shelley, Dixie, and I made a beeline for the shopping district. In Sacramento, if you want to go shopping, you head for a mall for everything you ever wanted and a lot you don't, all under one roof. Well, Japan has some places which might be comparable; there's one huge building, for instance, that is devoted entirely to electronics, but basically, we wandered stalls and shops of a different kind. There were narrow one- and two-lane streets lined with signs I could never hope to read. Behind those signs lay heaven!

"Lori," Shelley squealed, "you've got to see this!"

I dropped the silk blouse I'd been fondling and turned to the stack of playing cards Shelley was pointing to. Wait a minute—those were Chippendales' cards. Nude male dancers? In Japan? Sure enough, and Shelley bought them. The blouse I'd set down was outrageously cheap, but my eyes had already caught something I really wanted. There were dozens of watches lined up under a sheet of glass.

"Dixie, look. The answer to my dreams."

"I thought a rich pilot was the answer to your dreams." Dixie laughed and tried to compute the cost of a hand-beaded purse in American money.

"No, really," I said, "This watch can be set to different time zones. If we had one, we'd know at a glance what time it is wherever we're at. It's an electronic miracle. Jesus, the time we'd save calculating medication intervals alone would make it worth the price."

"Hey, let me see that." Shelley grabbed it. "I want two."

"Two?" Dixie raised both brows toward me in a great Groucho imitation. Shelley was definitely on a spending spree.

"I might lose one," Shelley replied defensively. "You never know."

Dixie and I looked at her skeptically.

"Well, you don't," she said smartly.

I started to make a clever comment but remembered the television I'd bought an hour earlier and decided, in this particular case, that silence was the better part of valor.

Eventually I ran out of cash, which turned out to be okay, because my arms could hold only so much and my legs could make only so many trips to and from the marketplace.

Then, on our last foray, this time in search of food, we saw an example of Japanese heritage that truly impressed me. Californians talk about the Gold Rush of 1849; the Japanese go back to 660 B.C., and that history is preserved everywhere. It seems almost to be an integral part of who and what they are. We saw some exquisitely dressed geishas, which I learned are professional dancers and singers, not prostitutes as so many of us thought. Being a geisha is a centuries-old profession, one they take obvious pride in. The women's enormous robes, carefully painted faces, and ornately styled hair made them living works of art. It was fascinating.

A few of us did a little sightseeing in between shopping and much needed naps. Japan really is a world apart. There's a Buddha surrounded by a halo of gold. It watches you with patient eyes and a raised palm. It's been there forever, and will remain there forever. That's Japan. State-of-the-art electronics right next door to almost three thousand years of tradition.

I liked it. I wanted to stay longer and learn more, but we had to get back to Hawaii.

Eight

Virginia Starr, Is That You behind Those Foster Grants?

"This is taking forever," Gary whispered over his shouler. "I mean, what do they think we're doing, stealing national treasures or something?"

Shelley twisted her lip to the side and shot Gary a mean look. "Shh. Keep it down, all right?"

"Jesus, Shell," Gary groused, "it's not like I have a geisha girl stashed in a TV crate or anything."

That must have been the straw that broke the Buddha's back or maybe the customs agent had a sister who actually was a geisha, I don't know. But a quick lift of a straight black brow, a few clicking sounds to his partner across the room, and we were all uncrating every single box and bag we owned. Nightgowns, panties, cosmetics strewn from one corner to the other. Spare flight suits, pressed and packed, were unfolded and pockets were searched and emptied. Jars of cosmetics got opened, sniffed, sometimes tasted. Twenty-five collections of newly purchased video gear and souvenirs were dismantled and carefully examined. It was one hell of a mess.

Accusing eyes latched onto Gary. "Cardinal rule number one," they seemed to say, "is never, never, never piss off the customs people."

And there, waiting to board and turning redder by the second was General Michael "Bomber" Basinger. It didn't look too good for Gary, and it didn't look too good for the 25th Air Evac.

Meanwhile, the inscrutable (?!) customs agents gleefully continued to turn our belongings and lives inside out.

Virginia kept a safe distance from Gary. He was, in her well-trained eyes, a felon of the worst ilk. Besides, the general was prime pickings, and Virginia was, and always will be, quite a picker. Or something like that.

A century later, when we were finally proven innocent of smuggling or whatever, we began our taxi down the runway. Virginia had managed to manipulate the seating so that she had ample access to her new target.

"General Basinger," she wrapped the fingers of her right hand around the dark fabric of his sleeve. "I'm so sorry that my crew caused you this terrible delay."

"It's quite all right, Virginia. These things happen sometimes," he said matter-of-factly.

Virginia? She already had him calling her by her first name? Boy, she did move fast.

"I assure you, sir," Virginia lowered her voice, deliberately being mysterious, "there will be changes made. My people are quite aware of how I feel about such things."

Her people? Heck, we thought we were the Air Force's people. Guess we and a few hundred thousand other airmen have been mistaken.

"By the way, General Basinger," she leaned forward, breathing close to his ear, "I've heard of you before. I'm impressed. Very impressed. I want you to know what an honor it is finally to meet you."

"Why, thank you." His voice mellowed and lost the steely edge he'd used earlier. "Do you fly this mission often? Perhaps we'll see each other again."

Cat and mouse. Twenty-four Air Evac crew members almost barfed.

Two hours later, Virginia was dangling her ample bosom a few millimeters from the general's face. "Excuse me, sir," she said softly, "I have to check again to see that everything is running smoothly. You know how it is when you're in charge."

I headed for the bathroom. By that time I was sure lunch would be history if I heard one more gurgle from Empress Starr.

I love flight suits. They have a billion handy pockets. As Virginia proved so effectively, they can be quite sexy and are extremely comfortable. But there is one tiny flaw in their design. Being all of one piece, a lady, by her very construction, must send them cascading all the way to the floor when she visits the restroom. The only alternative is to not visit the restroom. However, waiting all the way from Japan, for instance, until you reach Hawaii can be difficult. Twelve hours can be a long, long time.

Slipping the suit off my shoulders and letting it drop to below my waist didn't seem to be too much of an inconvenience until I surveyed the floor of the latrine area. I guess I should have checked it out before I sat down. You see, airplanes bounce sometimes, consequently, gentlemen miss sometimes.

How interesting, another ten full hours in a moist flight suit. I said, "Oh, darn. What a shame. Clumsy fellows," and pulled up my flight suit. I decided that when I hit Hickam Air Force Base, I would take a real good shower.

Virginia, I surmised, would need a shower as well. She was being so sweet to the general, she was downright sticky. It was, indeed, a long, long flight.

After awhile, the decision was made to cancel the

training exercise (we had only "pretend" patients made up of volunteer crew members). Everyone spread out and slept or read the rest of the trip. Shelley pulled out her Chippendales' cards and challenged me, Phil, Gary, and Dixie to a game of poker. I won two dollars and forty-three cents with two brunettes, a blonde in a G-string, and a pair of tight buns, but lost it all ten minutes later when I didn't manage to draw to the nineteen-inch biceps and snake-skin bikini. Gary had aces high—I had almost forgiven him for the customs fiasco in Japan. Que sera.

Still, it beat listening to Virginia entertaining the general, although some of us probably should have taken notes. As it turned out, the dear general wrote a letter of commendation citing the exemplary performance of Virginia Starr during that flight. She pretended to be important while the rest of us did the work and got the headaches, but she was the only one to receive an official pat on the back. Looked like while we were playing cards, old Virginia was playing the general.

Back in Hawaii, we had a problem with quarters. There were eight nurses who came in on that flight, and the billeting office at Hickam had only one hotel that had room for us. That was okay with us. We were hot, sweaty, and exhausted by then. All we wanted was a super fast shower and any available clean bed. We all agreed to go to the hotel billeting offered us.

Not all of Honolulu is on the beach, though, and Virginia seemed to think it should be. In Hawaii, a lot of the hotels have no doors leading from the street into the lobby. So you can just imagine seven exhausted women looking into an open doorway, mere feet from coveted cleanliness and rest, when the eighth suddenly comes to a complete stop and refuses to enter.

"Look, guys," Virginia began, and somehow I knew

we were in trouble again. "I know this great place right on the beach, and it's pretty much off season here now, so I'm certain my friends can get us in there."

"Your friends?" Dixie was too tired not to bite.

Virginia warmed to the subject. "Yes. It's just gorgeous there, I promise, and I know the managers. They've gotten rooms for me before. Think about it. We'll be right on the beach, so we can go out and sunbathe and sit on the patio drinking piña coladas. All of the men hang out around there, too."

"I don't want a man," Shelley sighed, "I want a bed. A big, empty bed."

"Won't it be a lot more fun to watch guys than stay in this old place?" Virginia was trying. One of the older nurses looked like she was warming to the idea.

"This hotel is not old, Virginia," Betty corrected. "The palm trees outside the lobby are old. The hotel is perfect. Now, let's all go in and get some sleep." She knew the rule about everyone staying together in case we were called and seemed determined to stick by it.

"Don't be a stick in the mud, Betty. Let's go to the beach."

"Look, we have to ship out for Tently tomorrow morning. We need our rest." Betty's voice took on an uncharacteristically hard edge.

Virginia ignored her comments and turned to the other nurses. "Who wants to go to the other hotel? Come on, it'll be great."

"I don't care where I sleep just so long as I sleep." Shelley flopped against the trunk of a giant palm and closed her eyes.

"Dixie?" Virginia shot a glance at Dixie, who seemed to be fairly easily intimidated at that point.

"Well," Dixie looked from me to Virginia, "I suppose

it's okay. I mean, if it doesn't take long."

"It will take long," Betty snapped. "Too long."

"Lori? You can jog on the beach in the morning." Virginia ignored Betty and tried her best smile on me.

I looked at my watch. We'd been standing in front of the hotel for close to an hour already, and all we'd done so far was argue when we could have been sleeping. I looked at Dixie. The trip had been hard on her, and Shelley was about to fall asleep standing up. The other new nurse stood quietly a few feet away from the group, obviously reluctant to take sides. I made up my mind right then and there that I'd had quite enough of Virginia Starr.

"No. We don't want to go." I grabbed my flight bag. "We are tired. We are going into this hotel right this minute and getting our rooms so we can go to bed."

Virginia glared at me. "Well, I guess you're making the decisions now, aren't you, Drew?"

"Whatever."

"I'm going to the other hotel," she snapped insolently.

I stared at Virginia. Did she really think she could intimidate everyone so easily? A dozen comments passed through my mind, but it would have been a waste of time, so I opted for a simple good-bye and stepped onto the tile walkway. When I headed for the check-in counter, Dixie, Betty, and Shelley followed me. I didn't know or care where Virginia finally landed, and after that, I made it a point never to fly with her again. The only exception was the jaunt back to California the next day. Even at that, we steered far clear of each other.

The trip from Hickam to Tently was to be another training flight. I had been assigned the task of flight nurse. It could have been an exciting time for me; it meant I would have enough time to qualify for flight nurse if I passed this last check ride. It was only slightly dampened by Virginia's pervasive cattiness and my sympathy for Dixie.

During briefing, I noticed that Dixie had been pulled from position and reassigned as a "patient." Since this was still a training flight we wouldn't be carrying any real patients, only Air Force personnel posing as such. My heart went out to Dixie. I could tell that she was hurt and disappointed. She tried to be game and act as if it didn't matter, but it did, and she couldn't hide the pain in her eyes.

The people who decide these things thought that she wasn't ready to continue, I guess. Perhaps they were right. She'd given a lot on the trip, and it had at times been long and harrowing. They do everything possible to make sure you're ready for any emergency, which means constant surprise cardiac arrests, hypoxia, respiration difficulties, and other critical situations. When the Air Force trains you to be an Air Evac nurse, you have to think fast and move even faster. And they felt Dixie needed more time to acclimate herself to the demands of the job; in addition, lack of sleep did not help.

She eventually made it through the trip, and when I got off the plane at Tently, Della laid her arm over my shoulders.

"Lori," she said, "you made it. You passed."

I was a full-fledged Air Evac nurse from that moment on. I knew there would be a formal presentation later and that I would have more tangible proof than just the feeling of elation that coursed through my veins, but I turned back toward the C-141 anyway. The big green lizard smirked. I smirked back and gave it a thumbs up. It was one hell of a ride, baby.

Nine

I Know I Have a Towel Around Here Somewhere

The Group had hardly disbanded once we were all safely through flight school and had been qualified. We more or less resumed where we'd left off as each of us returned to the nest. Once, Ginger managed to finagle her way into MCD position on a trip I was scheduled to be a patient.

We were headed to Oahu. I was listed as an ambulatory patient, but Ginger thought the nurse they were training should get a good dose of Murphy's Law. She walked over and nonchalantly tapped me on the forehead.

"Lori," she whispered, "you've just gone hypoxic."

I squinted my eyes, pretending to have difficulty focusing. My hands flattened themselves on my stomach, and I curled my lips into a nauseated grimace. My head flopped back against one of the wide strips of orange nylon webbing that composed my seat. I gave what I considered to be an Oscar-winning display of lightheadedness.

Ginger's eyes opened wide in appreciation. I'd done good. In fact, I'd done even better than she could have. I know this, because she promptly had me put on oxygen and strapped me to a stretcher, where I remained until the plane dropped gently down onto the concrete runway at Hickam. Ginger had a funny sense of humor. But then again, I would have probably done the same to her.

The two of us often got more and more insane as we spent time together. Some people just bring that out in a person, I suppose. We were quite a pair!

Ginger's real name was Gloria Heloise, but her family changed it to Ginger the moment her brown baby curls had started to transform into a fantastic mane of burnished red curls, which was probably all to the better. Knowing Ginger, she would have dumped Gloria Heloise and started calling herself Trixie if her family hadn't early on done her the favor of a more appropriate name. When I wanted to get her attention and she was ignoring me (which was often), I called her Gloria Heloise. It always worked. It also caused her to call me a lot of interesting things.

Once they removed my oxygen mask, I said, "Oh, Gloria Heloise, are you coming to the officer's club with me tonight?"

"No."

"Why not?" I asked innocently.

"No."

"There will be a lot of men and booze there, Gloria Heloise."

"No. I am going to be a model nurse and read select passages from *Gray's Anatomy* this evening." Ginger tried to look angelic. It was one of the very few things she was patently incapable of doing.

"Okay." I wrapped a blue shirt around my neck. It made me look like a World War II flying ace. Sort of. "Then I guess I'll go it alone. Off to Kalakaua Avenue."

Ginger eyes me suspiciously. "Kalakaua? Are you going to that seedy little bar that has those truly awful ventriloquist acts?"

"No."

"Why not?" Ginger asked carefully.

"Because there are more bars, more men, and more fun on the side streets."

"Then why did you say you're going to Kalakaua Avenue?" she persisted.

"Because," I put my cap on with a flourish, "it's the only name I can remember in that direction, and I don't have a car. I have to tell the taxi driver something, Gloria Heloise, dear."

"Wait a minute!" Ginger grabbed her flight bag. "I'm going with you."

"Quite," I replied.

"Shut up, fish face," Ginger chastised.

I did. Ginger, after all, was going to pay for the taxi. She just didn't know it yet. Besides, I couldn't very well leave her behind. She was an alto. I a soprano. Together, all we needed was a tenor and a bass to have a quartet.

We found them.

We'd been barhopping for an hour or two, when we tumbled onto the most perfect specimen of manhood in the Pacific. If Thor had been mortal, he would have looked just like this guy. I'm tall, but this Nordic blond towered a good six inches above me. All he had on was a T-shirt and Levis (God, I love hot climates!). Ginger started to drool.

"Back off." I positioned myself between her and Thor.

"I just want to touch him," Ginger sighed. "Just a little here, a little there."

I looked at her. "What a spectacle," I sighed.

Thor straightened his back. Was he going to leave?

My hormones propelled my feet forward until my chest was two point three inches from his biceps.

"Excuse me," I said. His eyes were blue. "You're the one I've been waiting for all my life."

Thor's mouth spread into a wide smile, revealing perfect teeth and dimples a woman could get lost in. He started to say something, but I turned and walked away.

It was good for me. I hope it was good for him.

Anyway, Ginger had found our tenor. Across the street, he insisted, could be found a bass. The four of us made a beeline down the streets of Hawaii, singing and dancing to the lyrics of any song we could remember and a few we couldn't. By the time we were back on Kalakaua, we'd been joined by three women and two men from nearby Fort De Russy. The nine of us converged on a small oasis of shopping called the International Marketplace. You could buy everything from shark's teeth to watch-sized video games at the Marketplace.

There was a tree right in the middle of all the little open air shops. It was supposed to be a magic tree, and a very pretty woman with hip-length gray-blonde hair told fortunes in a little wicker and grass hut at its base. Our group was diminishing to couples, and it was getting close to when Ginger and I had to get back to Hickam, but we stayed long enough to have our palms read.

The woman had very delicate hands with long, thin fingers. I felt like a giant as I laid my hand, palm up, in hers. She was so frail and had an almost wan smile. It didn't take much imagination to believe she really was privy to special powers. I'm not superstitious, but she told me a wonderful fortune.

I was to be getting someone and something new in my life. She said the person was going to change the way I saw and felt about the world. And there were to be a lot of animals in my future. It was very mysterious and, to my great surprise, later proved to be true. I wonder how she knew . . . or if she had a half-dozen pat answers that she gave to everyone. Did she read my future or did my future just fit what I remembered she had said? Sometimes I wonder about that.

Ginger didn't wonder much about her fortune. The tree lady told her that water was going to play an important role in her immediate future. So Ginger went back to the officer's club at Hickam and went skinny dipping. Ginger could be practical that way.

We thought the area was deserted. If it hadn't have been for some misplaced splashes, Ginger and I might have even thought we'd gotten away with it. But by the time we'd both surfaced, all we could see was the retreating figure of a young, broad shouldered man wearing a lime green swimsuit and carrying all our clothes.

"Uh, Lori," Ginger said, "do you think he'll come back?"

"I think so," I remarked, pleased by the calmness in my voice.

We watched him walk away. He didn't reappear.

"I guess we might as well finish our swim, huh?" Ginger gulped down the fit of giggles that threatened to overtake her.

A half-hour later, we were still in the pool and the mysterious stranger still hadn't come back. We snatched glances at the walkway every few minutes, but it was a lost cause. Eventually we had to swallow our modesty and climb out of the pool.

I lifted my chin high and vowed I would walk back to my quarters with dignity. Ginger was in favor of putting palm fronds over our faces as disguises. Fortunately for both of us and our future as Air Evac nurses, our night-caller had carefully laid our clothes on the ground just beyond the view from the pool. All our things were spread out to look as if we'd been lying spread-eagle on the ground when a mighty flying saucer had vaporized our flesh. It was a good joke, but I never found the guy in the lime green suit. Too bad. I have a few truly unique ideas for a payback.

Ginger and I made it back to the mainland the next day with our clothing and our reputations still intact. And she didn't put me through the hypoxia act again. (I secretly covet the notion that my acting was so far superior to hers that she didn't want the competition. She claims she was too involved with the green-eyed surgeon we were carrying to pay me any mind. The real truth, however, probably has something to do with a rather irritable passenger who also happened to be a general's wife.)

Bert had been having a little bit of trouble with an odd circumstance, too. He and I were scheduled to do a live mission (meaning that we would be carrying real patients) to Elmendorf Air Base in Anchorage, Alaska. When I met him at the Tently briefing, he was fit to be tied.

A good friend of his had been pulled from live flights and was only going to be allowed to take training flights with just enough frequency to stay qualified. It seemed that the Air Reserve Technician (ART) who was creating the problem had pulled Bert's friend because she was over the weight limit. Ordinarily this isn't a problem. If you were overweight you were put on the so-called fat-boy program and given time and incentive to get back within weight range. We all knew about the program; we all worked pretty hard to stay slim. The problem, the way Bert saw it (and to be honest, I agreed) was that the ART who was so busy forcing all his nurses to stay within their weight range was himself quite overweight and doing nothing about it.

It smacked of a double standard and, as a result, Bert wasn't in too good a mood over it. But there's one thing I can say about Bert. When he put on that flight suit, he left his other problems behind and became a hell of a nurse.

That's one of the reasons I liked him so much. He, like me, subscribed to the theory that taking things easy and looking at the humorous side can make a difficult job a lot easier. Sadly, however, this wasn't destined to be a congenial trip.

We expected the worst the minute we found out we'd be flying with an air crew from North Air Force Base. So far, the only contact either of us had had with North crews were all bad. They genuinely seemed to dislike Air Evac and were often difficult to get along with. My first meeting with a North pilot, in fact, had been an indication of things to come. He'd told me in no uncertain terms that Air Evac was a waste of time and he was sick of being assigned to do it.

This was a different pilot, but he and his cronies didn't show a lot of promise to be much better. Since we weren't allowed in the cockpit after take off, I went up there before hand to give the flight crew some information they'd be needing. One of the men up there turned a sourball face toward me, looked me up and down, and took his best shot at cutting down the dastardly flight nurse who was ruining his weekend.

"You've got the body of a twenty-year-old but the face of an old woman," he said in a nasty tone.

I looked at his squinty little cockroach face. I'd been prepared for some sort of sexist remark. It was a game these North fellows seemed to like to play. I knew he was just trying to get to me, but still it hurt. I didn't understand why they felt they had to be so cruel. Why does anyone ever say or do things that are so deliberately cruel?

Then I got mad. First of all, if he did think I had the body of a twenty-year-old, then, at forty, I could be damn proud of it. Second, I had enough boyfriends—both younger and my own age—who had told me I was pretty.

It was obvious that he wasn't too good a judge of beauty. I smiled sweetly and told him a catch phrase a neighbor girl had taught me when I was eight years old. Her mother was French. The phrase was in French and had something to do with a few interesting possibilities he could explore if he ever found himself in a flock of sheep.

Although I wouldn't have guessed it was possible, everything went downhill from there. One of our patients was a twenty-two-year-old man who had been in an auto accident two weeks earlier. He was being treated for head injuries. Shortly after take-off, he became unstable and developed ataxia. He had little control over his arms or legs. They were, in essence, as useless as noodles. Yet, every few minutes he would get up and go to the bathroom. Eventually we had to assign one nurse to do nothing more than watch after him. Because the ataxia made him clumsy, nothing in his range was safe from breakage. She really had her hands full.

It turned into a long and tiring flight. Even though it was twenty below zero outside, we were all very happy to set down on the concrete at Elmendorf. Three buses were due to arrive to take everyone on board to the medical complex. However, the patients' bus had broken down. Since we had to get them to safe quarters, we gave them our transport. As we were loading the patients on our bus, the flight crew climbed aboard their bus and left.

The entire medical crew was left standing in subzero temperatures waiting for the flight crew to send someone back for us. As evening moved in, with the wide expanse of flat ground it could blow over, the wind off the ocean sent the windchill factor plummeting. We were in danger of quite literally freezing.

We waited there for over an hour, which showed how important we were to the North boys. Thanks, guys.

Didn't anyone ever tell you that you're supposed to stay on board the plane until everyone is seen safely to their destination? The commander of our unit, who, fortunately, was on board thought so. At any rate, that was what the rules stated. He promptly wrote a disciplinary report on every member of the flight crew and sent it to headquarters.

The bad boys from North got into trouble. My, what a shame. The good part that came out of all of this, though, was that they treated us better and opened a line of communication from that time on.

Ten

Right in My Own Backyard

Most people spend their whole life just trying to get to Hawaii once. Now that I was an Air Evac nurse, I was able to fly there any weekend I wanted.

Finally. This was what I'd joined Air Evac for, and it was great. I'll tell you, there are worse things than spending every Saturday on the arm of a handsome pilot in paradise. So I took every mission I could. I didn't care if I was flying as a "patient" so another nurse could get checked out as a flight nurse. I loved it all.

The more I flew, the more I met pilots. Interestingly enough, my theory that all pilots come with wedding bands generally held true Yet, we had fun. It didn't matter whether we were in Idaho, Texas, Utah, Wisconsin, or Charleston, South Carolina. We'd go out to dinner together, go dancing, laugh, sing, and then wave goodbye as one or the other of us took off for home. Rarely would I see someone outside of the job. Except Alec.

He flew into my life with a dazzling display of *savoir-faire* and promptly wedged himself deep under my skin. He was a big, handsome man with a fast car, a love for airplanes, and a very understanding wife. Alec loved living life on the edge. He constantly searched for the next new adventure and embraced excitement and danger as he would a friend or lover. He was good for me in many ways.

But Alec was Alec. Not once did he make any bones about his being married or so much as even intimate that he wanted to be anything but. He came to me on those terms, "I'm an airline pilot. I'm an Air Force pilot. I'm married." That was Alec. He had no intention of giving any of those things up.

I didn't mind. I wasn't really looking for anything. I was divorced and not interested in remarrying. I also had a wonderful career that I didn't want to sacrifice to a personal relationship. I was at a point in my life where I was very comfortable with who and what I was. I'd found a way to live out some of my dreams. A "good friends but no strings attached" commitment was fine with me. Alec filled that need to a T.

We flew together frequently, and it wasn't long before dinner grew to affection. One night as we walked along the beach in Waikiki, I realized that I'd become the modern woman feminist magazines so often touted.

The setting sun had set the Pacific on fire, and the perpetual ocean breeze kept blowing wisps of hair across my face. I'd spent so much time beachcombing that my bare arms and shoulders had turned a deep golden bronze. I was in the best shape I'd been in for years, both physically and mentally.

Out of the corner of my eye, I could see Alec leaning against one of the small concrete picnic tables that sat under the palms. He was breathtaking. Sounds odd to say that about a man, I know, but it's true nonetheless. He was rubbing the tenseness out of his neck with the palm of one large, strong hand.

I thought, *This is every woman's fantasy: traveling all over the world, nights filled with laughter and parties, a successful career, a handsome man, and no strings. How long can it last?* Yet, I didn't fear losing it. My life was tangible. I didn't feel as if I was on a slide, careening out of control, but rather that I was a bird in flight, knowing exactly where I was going.

And it was good to have someone like Alec. It was nice to know that he felt enough at ease around me that he'd started coming to visit me at my house in Sacramento. Our relationship, though noncommittal, was beginning to flower. We would spend the nights together walking the beaches of Oahu, but the next day we'd fly back to Sacramento and go our separate ways. Except for intermittent meetings, it would stay that way until another Hawaiian sunset or need for company called. I was content. I didn't really need any more than that.

Then a friend of mine dragged me to one of her Toastmaster's club meetings. She said she needed moral support for the speech she had to give. She didn't tell me that there was going to be a former Air Force pilot there, too.

This guy was really funny. He stepped up to the lectern in a brown corduroy jacket that was literally ready to burst at the seams and flexed and preened through a myriad of muscleman poses. Then piece by piece and inch by inch the "muscles" were pulled free or fell out of the jacket until, at the end, he was a mild mannered insurance salesman. It was like from Superman to Clark Kent.

Within five minutes I was laughing my head off. Within a month, he was bugging me for dates. Within two months, I was bugging him for dates. And there went fate again, plucking me out of my own little world and smashing me face first into a new one.

He turned out to be not only funny, but also the most kind and gentle person I'd ever met. It didn't take long before Barry Chambers, budding comic and former pilot, became Barry Chambers, Lori Drew's best friend. I flew for two solid years, coming back each time to tell him about the good, about the bad, and about all the confusing and exciting things that happened to me. He became my port in the storm and my cabana on the beach. Good or bad, no matter what happened, I found myself anxious to get back to tell Barry.

I'd tell him about my trips and the people I worked and played with, and he always understood. He'd tell me about his time as a pilot and the new life he was trying to forge for himself. It became more and more important to me that he know and understand my life, where I was going and where I was coming from. He did.

I wasn't looking for a relationship. Didn't want one, in fact. Then one day I began to wonder if maybe it was time. I'd been assigned a two-week tour in Hawaii. I took off with my usual verve, expecting an incredible fourteen days of sunshine and laughter. I knew instinctively that I needed those two weeks to examine my relationship with Barry. Where was it going? Most important, where did I want it to go?

I left on my annual tour with those thoughts nagging in the back of my mind. Mia was due to meet me during the second week, and I was on call for any emergencies that might arise, so I knew I would be busy. I also knew there would be time for fun. There's always time for fun in Hawaii.

That Saturday, Shelley and Ginger flew in on an overnighter. Within minutes of their arrival, they stampeded my hotel room and forcibly hauled me off for a night on the town. (Okay. So they didn't have to force me, but I did make them ask nicely.)

They'd come in with the commander, who was one of the strangest birds I'd ever flown with. He could be great fun and had a much appreciated knack for looking the other way at really opportune moments. He also did this absolutely vicious imitation of another commander we all knew. Nicknamed the Boss, he was so full of himself there wasn't room for anyone else.

The four of us were having drinks in a sleazy little bar in one of the worst sections of Honolulu. Half of the men and a third of the women had tattoos, and there were more beer bellies and belching contests per square foot than I could have imagined possible. How and why we ended up there, I'll never know. Someone had thought it was a good idea, and everyone else was either too far gone or too hyper to be reasonable. So there we were, a little tribe of intrepid party-goers, solemnly discussing the relative merits of using the on-site lavatory facilities or trying to find, um, more sanitary accommodations.

Ginger felt that perhaps the ladies' room would be nicer than the mens', about which the commander had expressed some distaste in entering. There were, he said, strange noises coming from in there. We didn't question that. It seemed quite reasonable to us.

Maybe I'd spent too much time in the comfort-oriented Air Force, but I voiced a hope that the women's restroom would have those funny little sanitation donuts. Shelley agreed.

The commander sniffed audibly and flung himself gale force into a scathing rendition of our buddy, the Boss.

"There are no appreciable differences between female and male when it comes to cleanliness. A slob is a slob is a slob. And if either gender were to be more slovenly than the other, my money would be on the weaker sex. How can you possibly expect me to believe your facilities would be cleaner than ours?"

Shelley threw back the last of her rum and Coke, an

evil gleam in her eyes. "I think there's an important piece of information missing from our dear commander's repertoire. Don't you?"

Her gaze was locked on me. Uh, oh. I thought quickly. Was this a court-martial offense? I turned to Ginger. As I expected there was no help to be had there.

"Ladies," the commander sighed, still in the Boss mode, "you must remember that you are all members of a highly respectable and dignified profession."

We murmured amongst ourselves. He was right. We were.

"Okay," Ginger said, "we'll give you that."

"Right. Therefore, it would be unbecoming to you to pontificate on the relative merits of the appliances in the ladies' restroom." He smiled, obviously pleased with his choice of words.

"You're right, Commander. It would be silly of us to pontificate." Shelley placed herself low and to his right.

Ginger faced him, one hand resting on his opposite arm. "You do it so much better than we do, we wouldn't dream of trying to outmaneuver you."

"Okay, you guys," his eyes narrowed to tiny slits, "what are you up to? You never give up that easily."

"You know what they say," I laughed, "actions speak louder than words."

"Oh, shit!" His eyes bugged, and he started to run. Too late. Shelley swept a strong arm across the back of his knees at the same time Ginger put the full weight of her body against his chest. I caught him neatly with both arms as he fell.

Snatch and carry. In less than ten seconds, he was securely locked in the ladies' room. It was a major coup.

A muffled "Don't forget, I'm your commanding officer!" came from the other side of the door. Thing was, though, he wasn't putting too much effort into trying to break down the door. Must have been exploring.

One minute passed. Two. Three. Five. What was he doing in there, anyway?

Shelley opened the door a crack and peeked in. She couldn't see him through the narrow opening. The door creaked open another couple of inches, and we heard water running.

"Do we go in?" Ginger whispered.

I pushed the door wide and stepped inside. The commander, tall and dignified, was busy applying hand soap from the rusty wall dispenser.

"Why," he said flatly, "does the ladies' room not have a condom dispenser?"

The three of us cracked up just as a rather burly bouncer smashed through the door. "*Out!*" he bellowed, "All four of you."

We filed past, pretending to be repentant. The next day it was all over the base. I never was court-martialed. But I hope the statute of limitations for locking a commander in the ladies' room is up soon.

Less than two days later, on the 4th of July, the fun was over. I was "on call," and on my way to the beach, I got called and I found myself being shipped out on a live mission to transport a patient with gastrointestinal bleeding. I'd been up since 8:00 A.M., when I'd picked up my beeper. At that time, the senior nurse had okayed a trip to the beach, so I'd gathered food and scanned the map for a spot within the twenty-minute reporting distance.

It took less than five minutes, just long enough to get ensnared in a web of heavy traffic, for my beeper to go off. Phones? Nope. They're a vital part of life, to the point that we often take them for granted. But have you ever noticed how hard it is to find one when you *really* need it?

It seemed to take forever but was actually just minutes before I got out of traffic and into a phone booth. The news was bad. We had a fifty-year-old man with a history of GI bleeding who had gone on a drinking binge. His hemoglobin was eight, his hematocrit twenty-six. This man needed help—fast. I rushed back to base.

Back at the base, I dressed (quickly—nurses have little time for dawdling) and reported in. There would be me, two med-techs, and a flight surgeon in charge of bringing him back. Before leaving, we scrounged four units of blood, which wasn't easy to find. Ingenuity counts for a lot in Air Evac. Then it was off to Johnston Island.

Two hours later, we dropped down onto a bubble of earth no more than two miles wide and five miles long. A jeep sat on the macadam with little to serve as a backdrop; most of Johnston's buildings are underground. It took a short forty-five minutes to load the patient into the waist-high position of the litter stanchion and begin our taxi down the runway. I was strapped to the stanchion standing up throughout the flight, because the patient's blood pressure kept dropping and it needed to be constantly monitored.

I stood looking down on the man below me. From his records, I knew his name was Danny Groves, but I kept trying to talk to him and get him to give me his name. I needed to be able to assess his situation, and I knew the coherency of his answers could tell me a lot.

He wasn't able to focus enough to answer. His comments were all rambling, totally out of context. I began to worry, a large dry lump formed in my throat while my stomach twisted into knots. I took a deep breath and blinked a couple of times to relax the tension. Then I felt the plane leave the ground. The rumbling metal frame seemed to vibrate all the way to my core. The pressure of a standing take-off tended to unbalance me. Unconsciously, I thanked the Lord and the Air Force for the strong nylon webbing holding me to my patient's bedside.

"Danny. Danny." I talked to him quietly, hoping for some little response.

There was none. I attempted to take his blood pressure but got no reading at all. The plane was so loud, it was impossible to hear the faint beat of his heart through the stethoscope. I used my fingertips to palpate a reading. It was bad, so low as to be almost nonexistent. Through the entire flight, it alternated between dangerously low and unreadable. Even with the low hematocrit reading, the decision had been made to not give him blood yet.

Once the plane had leveled out, I called for Nancy, the med-tech, to give me a hand. She had been in Air Evac a long time and was very experienced. I really needed her to help me out and was relieved to have her and the other med-tech, Brad, make their way across the bumping plane. Still, Groves' body went cold and clammy as he lost blood pressure.

Air Evac went to work.

Danny's body spasmed in a couple of small involuntary jerks, and he began to heave. The fear left me, and all the years of training took over. Instantly, I grasped his jaw and tilted his head to the side so he wouldn't inhale his own vomit and choke.

"Nancy," I cried, just as two more capable hands reached toward Danny Groves. Calmly, efficiently, she took vital signs and organized the equipment we'd need to keep our patient alive. Brad had been one step ahead; he pulled what we'd needed from its storage space and set it out ready for her ministrations. I grasped his arm and, trying to hold the whole sky still, began an IV. All the while, the flight surgeon watched over us, giving orders, keeping track, and trying, then trying harder, to keep Danny Groves in the land of the living.

We did it. By the time we reached Hickam, he'd stabilized. I rode with him to the hospital in the ambulance, lights flashing and siren wailing, all the way to the hospital.

Danny survived that flight, but in a very real way, I didn't. Everything I'd left hospital nursing for had come back to haunt me. At times I had been in very real danger of losing my patient, and I found myself getting a little stressed because of it.

I was so disillusioned, I didn't know whether to scream or cry. Then Nancy came to me and asked if I would take her to the Fourth of July celebration downtown. She wanted to watch the ships come in and knew I had a car.

I really wanted to end the day on a pleasant note. I hoped so badly to find at least one glimpse of the high of nursing I'd known so intimately for so many years. We'd saved a man's life. I guess I just needed some reinforcement that it was good, that I could make it and not fall prey to burnout from too many tears over too many patients.

So I set aside my exhaustion and anxiety and drove Nancy through the tangled mass of traffic all of the way into town. I was more than happy to give her a ride. She'd worked hard, and I thought it would be nice to help her out. Yet, when we got there, she jumped out of the car, said a flat thank you as she walked away, and nothing more. That was the end of it. She hardly talked to me the rest of the tour.

She did talk to other people, though. I've never really been able to pinpoint what I might have done, but I know she must have harbored a lot of ill will towards me. Over the next week, she told a lot of people awful stories about me that weren't true but were only her interpretation of things. Fortunately, I'd worked with almost all of those people and they didn't believe what she said. But I didn't understand it. Maybe she felt that she could make more friends being the bearer of bad news. I think that for Nancy, this must have been the case.

I got back to my room, showered, and slid between the crisp, cool sheets. I was so tired. Every ounce of me cried out for rest, but I could sleep only fitfully. Early in the morning, I gave up and stepped out on the lanai to watch the sun come up.

I'd been in Hawaii for a little over a week. In that short time, I'd come full circle with my nursing, been subjected to petty infighting with the med-tech, and met a dozen handsome and willing men, none of whom I had the slightest interest in. I thought the Hawaiian tour would slowly fizzle to an end.

As usual, I was dead wrong.

Mila arrived on my doorstep with a big smile and a fragrant lei. The second she laid eyes on me, she knew I was having some problems.

"On call?" she asked as she draped the lei over my shoulders.

"Nope." The flowers smelled so good, a little ray of pleasure. Funny how something that simple can make such a big difference. "God, Mila, it's so great to see you."

Mila smiled and then laughed. "Oh, I know that! Poor thing. You look tired. What you need is a little relaxation. Didn't anyone ever tell you that Hawaii is paradise? Why aren't you out having fun?"

"I don't know. Just a little stressed out, I suppose."

Mila lifted a brow. "Yeah, I heard. That med-tech is really letting you have it, huh?"

"You mean you've already heard?" I flopped on the bed in disbelief. "What's she doing? Taking out ads in the newspaper?"

"Nah," Mila started rummaging through the closet. "You know how people talk. Actually, everyone is getting more than a little tired of listening to her garbage. She's a bitch, Lori, and everybody knows it. Ignore her."

A white linen jumpsuit flew through the air and wrapped itself around my head.

"Here," Mila said, "wear this. It's sexy but not enough to make me look like a Little Bo Peep."

"You don't look like Little Bo Peep."

"Around you I do."

I looked at the pastel pink-and-white striped sundress Mila had on. Spaghetti straps, fitted bodice, long shapely legs under the full skirt. Nope, no one was going to mistake her for Bo Peep.

I wore the jumpsuit anyway.

Hickam was right next door, so all the marines from Pearl Harbor would drop over to the officer's club to get a little R&R on Friday nights. Which meant that the club was always a little rowdy. This Friday wasn't any different.

Mila was great company, and before I knew it, Nancy and the disappearing surgeon were both just faint memories. A few drinks later, they weren't even that.

A large group of marines wandered in, each one in a different T-shirt. This, of course, required a detailed study of the men and the shirts, as well as a discussion of the relative merits of both.

"People," I said with authority, "all wear their own identity."

"No, they wear whatever they own that isn't dirty." Mila had a point, but I considered it only superficial.

"On the surface only, Mila. I mean, look at those men. There. What about the one in the Mickey Mouse shirt? See how he's clowning around?"

Mila waved a hand in the air. "Lori, you have a white jumpsuit on. It doesn't mean that you're a parachutist for the KKK."

"Get serious." I pushed the hair back out of my face and tried to look scholarly. "What about the Mouseketeer?"

"His mom probably sent it to him."

"Mothers don't give their grown sons Mickey Mouse shirts." I said logically.

"Maybe one of his ex-girlfriends gave it to him." Mila snickered. "Maybe she was trying to tell him something."

"Okay, I'll agree to that. Especially since it only goes to prove my point." I snaked out my arm and grabbed the wrist of one of the marines as he tried to twist past us. "Now here. Look at this. This is exactly what I mean. You see, he's wearing a red T-shirt. Red is a strong, flashy, courageous color. Are you strong, flashy, and courageous?"

The marine laughed and looked at Mila. "Sure. Why not."

"See what I mean?" I said and jerked Mila around the booth to make more room. "Sit down, um . . . "

"Jake." He said and sat next to Mila.

"See? Am I right, or what? His name is Jake. A perfect red name. You're extroverted, too right?"

Jake looked at me, "Why aren't you wearing red?"

"Because of Bo Peep." I motioned toward Mila.

Mila smiled wanly. "We must forgive Lori. She's lost too many brain cells due to lack of oxygen."

"Jake?" I pressed.

"Yes?"

"Being a true wearer of red, would you save a damsel in distress?"

"That depends," Jake answered, but didn't take his eyes off Mila, "on the damsel in question."

"Oh," I said. Sometimes it takes awhile, but sooner or later the light always dawns. "Gee, guys, I have an early call. Have to run."

"Lori," Mila quirked her brows into twin question marks. "How are you doing?"

My friend Mila. She had an absolutely gorgeous marine drooling all over her chest, and she was still worried about me.

"Since I can walk back to quarters from here, I'll be fine." I smiled. Yes, I knew I would be. Some things had suddenly become very clear in my mind. "In fact, I feel great."

Jake held out his hand. "Nice meeting you, Lori. Take it easy. Okay?"

"Sure," I replied happily. "Oh, and Jake?"

"Yeah?"

"The color pink," I pointed to Mila's sundress, "means affection and femininity."

"Thank you, Lori." Mila commented dryly.

She couldn't have been too angry, though. She ended up marrying Jake. And I was proven right . . . again.

In fact, it was an odd thing that happened that night. It looked like it was going to be nothing more than another night out. Men, women, games. But as I walked back to my hotel, I realized something very important. None—not even one—of the men I'd met in those two weeks did anything for me. I didn't care about them. I didn't need them. I didn't want them.

What I wanted, and what I did, was to go home to

Barry. I knew from that moment on that BC, as I'd come to call him, could be a part of my life. All I could think about was getting back to Sacramento and telling him about my experiences. And that felt good. It felt very, very good.

I'd spent all that time flying all over the world, never really caring about or looking for a relationship, thinking that Air Evac was all I wanted. And then there he was. Cupid zapping me when I least expected it. And not on some far-off corner of the globe, but right there, in my own backyard.

Eleven

I Like the Idea of Feeling Comfortable for the Rest of My Life

Barry and I wanted our wedding to be something very special, something representative of the lives we led, the feelings we had for each other, and the hopes we had for our future. It took a lot of planning and, quite often, looking at ourselves with a sense of humor, but in the end we had exactly what we wanted.

Because horses had always been such a passion of mine, I thought it would be nice to have them a part of our wedding. So BC and I literally rode to the altar. We braided ribbons in the long mane of Barry's mount, matching them to the blue saddle blankets we used. I was to ride Topah, my pride and joy, the horse I'd bought with my nursing school money.

Everything was carefully planned to misplace time. Slowly we wove the horses through the trees and onto the outdoor arena, where we would be taking our vows. We both felt strangely at home in our clothes. Barry could have passed for a dapper Bat Masterson, and I relished the ease and presence of my vintage blouse, hat, and riding skirt. As we neared the arena, I could hear small snatches of Pachelbel's "Canon" playing in the background and see, here and there, a glimpse of the blue and white ribbons encircling the fence. Closer still, the cerulean plaid of our ushers' shirts and mauve rustle of my maid of honor's dress peeked through the pines.

At the gate to the arena, Barry dismounted and walked to the lattice-and-vine covered altar. Behind him, I followed, first at the side of a dear friend, then on the arm of my father. It was the last few steps to a whole new life for me. My maid of honor Mila handed each of us a glass of mellow almond champagne. I held it carefully, watching through the shimmery lace of my veil the man who would very soon be my husband.

Barry smiled and raised his glass, ready to speak. "Ladies and gentlemen," he began, "I propose a toast to Lori Drew. Now, some of you probably don't know the first night I met Lori, she came in and she told me what a wonderful person I was. And several minutes later she came up and said, 'I'm sorry. I had you confused with someone else.'"

It sounded funny, but it was true. Little did I know what it would bring.

BC paused and looked thoughtful. "Now, I thought I had gotten all that ironed out, and a few weeks ago I went and I picked up the wedding invitations. And she mailed a few of them out. And I said, 'By the way, am I invited to this wedding?' and she said, 'Well, yes. Why?' And I said, 'Well, because my name isn't on that invitation.' And if any of you got an invitation for Lori Drew and Bartholomew Lee Chambers, I have no idea who Bartholomew Lee is, because my name is Barry."

As our friends laughed, I thought, *This is right. So special.* It seemed to fit that BC and I would begin our life together on a happy, laugh-filled day.

Barry looked at me. "But I found over a period of time knowing this lady," he continued, "that there's just one thing about her, that being with her I just feel comfortable. And I decided that I like the idea of feeling comfortable for the rest of my life. And that's why I'm here now."

All our guests cheered. And I knew, without a doubt, that I not only loved this man, but that I cherished him as well.

Barry raised his glass in a toast. "To Lori Drew."

The world blurred, and a moment later, the minister's voice wrapped some truly special words in a silken cocoon. "I now present Mr. and Mrs. Barry Chambers." And I was married to Clark Kent, Superman, my friend, my confidant, the person who anchored my past, shared my present, and promised my future.

Afterwards, all our friends gathered on a haywagon and rode to the reception. Champagne flowed, people laughed, and I decided that *this* was the best party I'd ever been to. No doubts whatsoever.

It was several months later that BC and I got our honeymoon.

My annual tour with Air Evac was due, and I drew Elmendorf, Alaska. Barry and I thought, "Well, two weeks in Alaska. Why not?" So we set it up that I would go on my tour as usual and BC would fly up to join me during the second week so we could have a honeymoon. It promised to be a very special trip, and I was more excited than I'd been in a long time.

I landed at Elmendorf AFB in Anchorage on a day that was designed for magic. Alaska is . . . majestic. You can see forever, and the sky is so blue, you feel as if you can reach up and touch it. Elmendorf is in a little valley. As you face one side, gray waves crash in from the Pacific Ocean by way of Cook Inlet, and to your back are snow-frosted mountains that climb to dizzying heights. Everything, absolutely everything, is green, blue, or white.

Anchorage is something few people expect, but I

would guess a lot are ready for. It's small, as cities go, and a wonderful surprise for this Californian—almost void of congestion, both from traffic and people. I was in heaven!

For the whole two weeks I was there, I was on call twenty-four hours and off twenty-four, which meant that I would have plenty of time to see the sights and have fun. First, though, I needed to spend some time with my crew. There were a lot of behind-the-scenes tasks that needed to be carried out in Air Evac. Things no one thinks about or notices—unless they aren't done; if they aren't taken care of, the whole system can (and probably would) come to a complete halt in a jumble of confusion.

The crew and I all put in time at the detachment setting up our equipment and taking inventory to be certain we'd have everything we would need if we were called. There aren't a lot of things more frightening than knowing you could have saved a life, relieved some suffering, or helped someone if only you'd had the right equipment. Add to that the anxiety of realizing you're the one who left that one important piece of gear behind, it's easy to see why we put time and double time into making sure we were prepared for almost anything.

We also got to spend a day going through a new facet of survival training.

"What do you do if you crash in the Arctic?" two training officers asked. And since they didn't like my med-tech Greg's suggestion that we pray for a heat wave, we went over and over Arctic survival and rescue techniques.

Interesting, to say the least. I think I would have preferred crashing over Texas, when you get right down to it. (Actually, it's my express opinion that planes should stay up until I want them to come down. Sadly, fate doesn't always agree. I always have and always will get very nervous when a pilot says, "Uh, oh.")

On one of the first days I had off, I approached some of the crew and asked them if they wanted to go to a place up in the mountains I'd heard about that rented horses. If there was one thing you could always depend on from an Air Evac crew, it was that at least a handful were game for just about anything. I immediately had four volunteers.

I've learned a lot over the last few years. For instance, the stories you were brought up on about the Air Force and the Wild Blue Yonder are true. And the tales you've heard about wild and woolly Alaska are also true. None of us could believe the Mother Lode Ranch when we got there. It was like stepping back to the 1800s. Unless you were fond of dogsleds, snowmobiles, and frostbite, the lodge was unreachable in the winter. So it remained open only during the summer months.

It was easy to see why it was so inaccessible. The Mother Lode Ranch was nestled in a crook in the mountains. Even with your feet firmly rooted in one spot, a cavalcade of incredible sights cropped into view from every corner. The deep winter snow and fertile ground provided fodder for miles and miles of lush greenery, all the more fascinating for its unbelievably diverse forms. Then, as if Mother Nature felt a need to punctuate her comment, a huge jumble of gray rock would suddenly burst from the foliage-covered mountainside. Right near the ranch's hitching posts, two stone-maddened creeks converged to form an even angrier river. The lodge itself had been built further up the slope and was reached by a long C-shaped staircase. It marked the last vestige of civilization before entering gold mining country. There were, in fact, several of the old mines still being quarried.

A wonderfully witty woman ran the Mother Lode when she wasn't busy being a schoolteacher in town. With little provocation, she and her husband, an Alaskan congressman, would weave fascinating tales of Alaskan life. Like many others, she'd moved from southern California to Alaska to get a teaching job. Unlike a lot of her compadres, she'd immediately fallen in love with the land, the people, and the lifestyle. Yes, she agreed, winters were hard. Sometimes unbelievably so with the short days, cold temperatures, and unrelenting snow. But it was something you learned to adjust to, and neither she nor her husband could imagine living anywhere else. Alaskans, I discovered, like their state, are a hardy and independent lot.

The whole atmosphere was totally different from anything most of us had ever encountered. Everything was just kind of laid back and relaxed. It was almost as if the people there knew the land has been there for millions of years and will be there for another million, so why rush? Why worry? Sit back, relax. Make yourself at home.

And we did. We rented horses and wandered for awhile around the mountains, exploring the gaps and ridges that all offered up a new and interesting adventure. As the temperature dipped, we headed back to the lodge and gathered in the warm dining area for shared bowls of chili and Paul Bunyan-sized hamburgers. It was somewhat disappointing to have to climb back in the car for the drive back to the base, but all play and no work gets you fired. So we opted for shopping and jogging in Anchorage.

Most of the time there I just sat and bided my time, waiting for BC. The day he was due to come in, I enlisted the aid of another Air Evac nurse. Now, there's one thing I really love about my husband—he knows a good joke when he sees one. Or should I say—when he's the butt of one?

Good old BC climbed aboard an airplane on a warm and inviting California morning and headed for cold old

Alaska, and he was really truly happy about doing it. Why, you ask, would an otherwise perfectly sane man be thrilled about leaving tennis shoes and sunblock SPF24 for long johns and frosty earlobes? Well, it was going to be our honeymoon, remember. Instead of being greeted by a snowstorm, he was going to step off the plane in Anchorage and fall into the waiting arms of his new bride!

So he got on the plane. Next stop, Alaska.

I drove to the airport. Next stop, my hiding place behind a huge post, completely out of sight of disembarking airline passengers.

BC got off the plane.

Oh, sad faces. Where was his beloved bride? *The one who promised she would be there! The one who was going to keep him from being all alone and lonely in the least populated state in the whole country!*

I pointed him out to my friend, who then took a lot of great photographs of the metamorphosis BC's face went through as he traveled the road from "Hi, Lori, it's me!" To "Lori, are you here?" through to "Oh, my God, I'm stranded in Alaska . . . I can't find my wife . . . what am I going to do now?" "The thought of her not being here never entered my mind. What if something happened to her? Who do I call? Where do I go? I am not having fun . . . this is no way to start a honeymoon."

It was great, but I couldn't hide any longer; the pain on his face was just too much. A joke is one thing, but a joke that turns into pain is another. I jumped out and ran to hug and kiss him and all was forgiven.

Our good fortune (or good planning!) was that I wasn't on call that night. So we gathered ourselves together and headed for one of the outdoor barbecues the locals put on regularly. Alaskans really know how to eat. It must be the cold or something, but they have a penchant for great food in enormous quantities. I don't know how anyone could live there and not weigh a ton. These barbecues were honest-to-goodness feasts.

A certain kind of clarity comes with the mere simplicity of crisp autumn air blended into shimmering starlight, gunmetal gray woodsmoke, and an ever-shifting array of festival lanterns. The round-bodied scent of salmon and ribs charbroiling over open fires permeated the entire area. Before long, we found ourselves cuddled together over smoked salmon, oblivious to the cold in our cocoon of starlight and moondust. The honeymoon had just begun.

It still hasn't ended.

Later, we spent a very cozy night getting to know each other again and spent all the next morning doing something you got to do blessed little of in the Air Force—we slept in. Everything was sunny and bright for me during those days. I had the most wonderful feeling of having my life in perfect sync. I was young, in love, traveling all over the world, the top in my career field. And I was on my honeymoon in the jewel of North America, Alaska.

BC, being a pilot, thought we could rent a plane and see some of the country from one of our favorite places, the sky. After getting checked out (a prerequisite for renting a plane), BC and I took off to see Alaska from a new vantage point. From God's point of view, mankind has done little to change the face of the forty-ninth state. When you're flying over her, you can see forever. Looking down, all you see is nothing.

Absolutely, unequivocably nothing.

No pockmarks of overpopulation.

No gouges cut with bulldozers and dynamite.

No volcanic tufts of man-made smog.

No razored battle scars attesting to the conflict between man and nature.

Nothing.

Just pristine wilderness that goes on as far as you can see and beyond. The last enchantment, the land in Alaska.

Sadly, I wasn't able to spend much time enjoying it. The air turbulence was kind of weird and, veteran flyer though I was, I became increasingly airsick. The worst of it was that the mountains forced us to higher elevations, yet the higher we flew, the worse the turbulence. BC must have forgiven me for scaring him at the airport, because he kindly dropped to a lower altitude and found a quaint little airport and set the plane down for our lunch.

Next to the airport was a dense forest of birch trees. It provided the perfect haven for a gracious pilot and his green-gilled wife to unwind, stretch their legs, and down a picnic. The thin white trunks of the trees spun a tight web, a natural maze one had to be careful in or become irretrievably lost. We wandered around, but not too far. It was far too beautiful a place to take for granted or test. So we sat and ate our lunch, marveled at this fascinating new corner of earth's magic, and pinched ourselves that we were really there and our lives were gliding along in such a special and precious way.

After a leisurely walk through the thicket, we took off again and searched out a lake with a nearby airstrip. It was an attractive splash of cerulean nestled amongst pine trees and deep wheat-colored meadow grasses. A long walkway of hastily tacked boards led to the water's edge. More than one person had pulled a grandaddy of fresh water salmon out of its depths. We strolled and even stopped for a short nap but eventually had to make a beeline back to the airport. An airshow was being held the day we decided to go sightseeing, and it promised to be a taxing endeavor to land the plane amongst the teeming masses. But BC, with his skills in flying and his command of the control panel, was able to ease us in quickly and without mishap. Just another day in the life of a pilot. And even with the earlier air turbulence, I didn't once lose my lunch. Hey, sometimes one has to just say, "All right! Great day!"

I could barely wait to take BC to the Mother Lode. I rather liked the idea of blazing a trail where there was nothing even remotely resembling civilization for miles. I couldn't help but marvel at the strange and different faces my world had taken on. I'd been in cities populated by millions of people, and here I was dodging moose, reindeer, and a rather ornery and gluttonous Alaskan brown bear just to get to ride a horse.

I'd heard talk about the ferocity of an angry mother bear. With that firmly planted in mind, we pretended to be patient. Pretend is about all you can do. Going out *to* dinner and waiting for a table is one thing; when you're being sized up *as* dinner, patience is a definite, if not overly tranquil, virtue. So we waited. And she waited. And we hoped she preferred not to take her meals out of the can. And she hoped (I'll swear to this in a court of law) that we'd get out of the car so she wouldn't have to worry about breaking a nail on the aluminum window flashing.

The bear eventually granted us passage, and we covered the last few miles to the lodge. When we got there, our horses were waiting. They'd saddled up a pinto for BC, but I don't know why, I thought that maybe he would prefer one of the other horses. But Barry insisted on the pinto. He claimed it was two-toned, like a good old Ford. I thought about pointing out that his Ford was a Mustang and solid blue, but I knew Barry, and I knew that if pressed for an explanation, I would probably spend the rest of the afternoon trying to figure out what exactly he'd said. You don't argue with BC's logic. He rode the pinto.

Barry and I found our guide, then packed the saddlebags, tightened the cinch, and headed out into the wilderness, not knowing what to expect. This, I discovered, is a pretty safe assumption when you're dealing with Alaska.

Two miles down the road, we ran into a herd of buffalo. They couldn't care less that we were successful professionals slowly, but efficiently, climbing our way up the career ladder. They thought, in fact, that "where the buffalo roam" was a government mandate granting them sole and proprietary use of the wilderness. I looked at the muscles fluidly stretching beneath the heavy umber coats. The largest buffalo of the group obliged by turning his face to me, exposing a flat forehead matted with a thick thatch of curls.

He didn't look happy.

And our horses were starting to get skittish. I was starting to get skittish.

Our guide helped a lot. "Better take it easy here," he said. "Don't want them to attack us."

Gee, thanks, I thought. That really put me at ease.

Dodging and weaving, we made our way around the perimeter of the herd. The horses were hot, sweaty, and pretty excited. Fortunately, all three of us were experienced riders, so we were able to handle them well enough to get safely past the buffalo. I think, though, that the big one memorized my face and is still waiting for me.

As we traveled further down the road, the terrain worsened, becoming steep and rocky. It was easy to see that this was a relatively seldom used area. In many places it looked as if we were breaking new ground. The only signs of humanity were the things we'd brought in.

Then, seeming to pop right out of a wall of granite, there was an inverted U of rough hewn timbers holding open the gaping mouth of a mine.

Curious, as we were, we stopped and had lunch and pondered if we should or shouldn't enter the mine. Our guide told us that we could get shot if caught in the mine. So it was unanimously decided to venture no further than the front entrance. The buffalo, after all, still had our number, and the bear was probably back on the road licking her chops. The last thing we needed was a miner deciding to defend his claim with a double-barreled shotgun.

After lunch, we pressed the horses on up the trail, the only sound that of clopping hooves on leaf-covered ground until, eventually, passage was made impossible by the outcroppings of rocks and trees.

Turning back, we looked down on the mountain we'd ascended. All around us nature was decked out in her finest, a beauty so complete, it literally took our breath away. Below us a verdant valley anchored the snow-capped ridges and mountain peaks. Glacial ice reflected the sun's bronze glow with here and there wide and erratic ribbons of cinnabar and cadmium. To the side and below the cliff we were perched on, a swiftly moving white-water river sliced a vengeful path of rocks and crashing sprays. Crowning it all was a velvety sheet of sapphire sky. It was so magnificent as to make one feel both bigger than life and small and humble at the same time.

It was not the kind of place that was easy to leave, but by then, we were all pretty tired, cold, and hungry. Sun-warmed afternoons can settle in at seventy degrees, but with each change of scenery, so can there be a change of comfort. It was getting late, and no matter how warm the day, nights could bring a definite chill. So we headed back to the lodge for a huge serving of the World's Greatest

Homemade Chili. (I know that almost every chili house on the face of the earth claims this, but, honestly, in this case, it's true.) After consuming a hefty portion of chili garnished with fresh onions, cheddar cheese, and homemade bread, we sat back and downed a cool beer. A real lumberjack's dream.

Oh, yes, Alaska is the land of beautiful shores, green terrain, hot chili, and adventure worth experiencing. It's one of the few places remaining where you can feel the earth, wind, and sky. The last frontier, Alaska is what America used to be like—when it was pure, when you could see forever.

Twelve

Just a Heartbeat Away

I was on call. The rules when on call were simple. Don't get far from base because the beeper could go off any minute, and don't drink any alcohol because—right—the beeper could go off any minute. BC and I decided, okay, then, let's go jogging.

Texas has a way of saying, "Hey, look at me, I'm the greatest." To tell you the truth, Alaska probably has a better claim to the statement. Even the golf courses are out of the ordinary. We found ourselves jogging around a lush spread of perfectly manicured grass tickled on the edges by a babbling brook and serene woods. It was a wonderful run that primed us for dinner in a fancy restaurant in town.

So after having this wonderful, wonderful week so far, we decided, "Let's keep it going. We, after all, might never get this chance again." And so we did. Dressed and ready, we ate a gourmet fish dinner. Then I made a little mistake.

Barry, convinced I wouldn't be called to duty, talked me into a glass of white zinfandel. A little white wine never hurt anyone who kept herself firmly planted in a well-cushioned chair in a fine restaurant. But in my case, guilt immediately set in. What, I imagined, would happen if I had to fly? I could get sent home, and not with a bouquet of roses, either.

I still felt a little giddy from the wine when we decided

to get a piece of rhubarb pie a la mode and cappuccino at a fantastic pastry shop called, for reasons I'll never know, California Roll. (This was an interesting thing I discovered in my travels; when and where you least expect it, someone will transport little chunks of the world to the most incongruous places. An Arizona cactus will be painted on the side of a tavern in Oregon, a palm tree will be the logo for a theater in Michigan, a developer will call himself Snowcap Realty in Bakersfield. Makes one wonder. . . .)

Anyway, BC loves rhubarb pie, and he also doesn't hear as well as I do (no, that isn't a non sequitur, really), so I was quite surprised when he told me my beeper was going off. I didn't believe him at first, but he wouldn't have stopped chewing that great pie if he hadn't really thought he'd heard something. So I relented and searched out a phone to call the base.

Sure enough, Sergeant Juarez had been paging me.

"We have a patient on Shimea with a head injury, and they need an Air Evac there right away." The sergeant continued, "He's unstable . . . you have twenty minutes to get back here to the base. Make it fast."

I stared at the phone, remembered the seemingly innocent glass of wine, said, "Oh, shit!" and tried to keep my stomach from smashing into the polished oak flooring.

"BC, we've gotta get back to the base. I've got a live Air Evac mission.

"Oh Christ," he replied. "Wouldn't you know it!"

It was about 6:00 P.M. We left our rhubarb pies behind and hurried back to the base. We were there within minutes, and while I was dressing and packing, BC made me some coffee. It wasn't because he thought I wanted any, but he figured, and I agreed, that it would help cover up the wine on my breath.

I barely got to the dispensary within the allotted twenty minutes. Sergeant Juarez quickly briefed us on what was to come.

I was designated MCD, and the other nurse and techs basically all worked together with my senior tech acting as charge tech. The other nurse was from the Nebraska group. Her name was Elise; she was trained as a psych nurse as well as being the dean of nursing at the University of Nebraska. I couldn't help but think, *Well, this is going to be interesting.* As God is my witness, I didn't realize then how interesting it was going to get. In addition, they had paratroopers fly along just in case.

That was it. Paratroopers. Two nurses. A flight surgeon. Med-techs. All on our way to Shimea to help a twenty-six-year-old patient with a head injury. In the five hours it took us to get there, we covered all the possible scenarios we could come up with. As expected, we set up duties for each person, planned loading configurations, how and what we would do to help the medical unit on Shimea care for this patient, who was already in cardiac arrest and receiving CPR.

It was two o'clock in the morning before we taxied down the runway and sprinted to the dispensary, where the patient had finally stabilized. After being briefed by the Shimea crew, the decision was made to transport a very pale, but functioning on his own, Airman Sloane back to Anchorage.

When the med-tech turned him over to put him on the transport board, John Sloane's heart stopped, the cardiac monitor flattened to a hard, unforgiving line.

All our minds instantaneously went into overdrive. One med-tech began chest compressions while the other clasped an ambulbag to the patient's face. On the doctor's orders, I prepared and administered drugs. Drugs that should have helped John Sloane breathe again, helped his heart to beat again. Minute after minute ticked by as we all worked in unison. Close to an hour passed, and aching backs and shoulders were relieved of the unending up and down movements of CPR. I stared down in the face of this very pale, very quiet young man and felt the acrid smell of fear rise in my nostrils.

I rhythmically moved my flattened palms up and down on his chest, praying that the very desire bashing the insides of my ribcage could be forced from my body into his by the sheer strength of my need for him to live. "God . . . damn . . . you . . . " The words spewed from my mind, only to be trapped in the constriction of my throat, never to be heard by those men and women surrounding me. "Don't you dare die! I won't let you! I won't! I won't!"

I don't know why it so surprised me that my mind had suddenly started working on two levels. While I automatically measured the depth and timing of the chest compressions, I, at once, watched it all in a state of limbo. God help me, I didn't want the young man below me to die. I wanted, desperately needed, to see him smile, hear him laugh, watch him live. He wouldn't. And I, after ten challenging and fulfilling years of caring for the critically ill, after even more years in which I taught nursing, and three great wonder-filled years of being an Air Evac nurse, I died with Airman John Sloane. Thousands of miles from nowhere, on the farthest island of the Alaskan chain, it was over. For both of us.

I sucked air between my lips and pressed my front teeth hard in on themselves. John Sloane had transferred to the Air Force base on Shimea a week earlier. It didn't seem long enough for something to happen to take his life. It was a tragic and unfortunate accident, and totally unfair.

As he lay there, so young, so still—so dead—a sensation of intense desolation swept over me. The bitterness of cold despair crept into the very corners of my soul and lay there, a festering wound robbing me of all power. I closed my eyes, willing away the aching torment that had locked its unforgiving grip on my heart. I was a nurse. I had to handle this, as I had done hundreds of times before.

I tried. I had desperately tried to help save John Sloane, and couldn't.

Outside the dark caves of my mind I heard Elise gently coaxing the others into going through the steps necessary to close the book on Airman Sloane. My mind closed, too. I knew that as the charge nurse my job was no longer to remain with the patient but to make other preparations. I had to deal with that.

Elise prodded me toward the door, telling me to go to work on the reams of paperwork the government required for everything, even death. She was a saint in a flight suit. I'd never been so grateful to have a psych nurse around in my entire life. This was her realm, her area of expertise, so I went with it, letting her take over.

I stepped outside, so thankful to be able to leave that little room that an involuntary shiver racked my body. I tilted my face to the clear, cool sky. I needed to get myself together. I had paperwork to fill out and get approved, a dozen tasks to perform. It was my job to get the necessary clearances so we could take John Sloane back to Alaska. So he could go home for the final time. Christ! He was too young to bury. Too young. Too young.

All the years of study, of practice and caring, of trying and sharing, and I still hadn't been able to save him. The grief rushed through me with hurricane force. My ears roared, my eyes burned, and my mouth throbbed an echo to the pain in my shoulders.

And I cried.

It took three hours to get the paperwork approved to transport Airman Sloane back to Alaska. Even then, it was only because the flight surgeon had enough pull to rush it through. Our small group loaded the silver coffin into the belly of the C-130. We would spend the next five hours moving through time and space, on our way to complete our lives. Things Airman Sloane would never do again.

So we listened to the sounds of the plane and the beat of our hearts and waited for those interminable minutes and hours to tick past. We were prisoners of our own thoughts. It was a long flight, and I had time to do a lot of soul-searching about Air Evac, about where I was at and what was going on. I needed to use the restroom, but to do so meant stepping on John Sloane's coffin. There was no way to avoid it. Miserably I lay back on my bunk and wished I could be somewhere, anywhere else.

Then I realized that I didn't want to do this anymore. Air Evac had given me some wonderful times. I'd met some great people and gone to a lot of exciting places. But the reality of the job was that I was still a nurse, even though I had, as Commander West said on graduation day, angel wings on my back. I'd spent too many years in critical care and seen too much. Too many times I had to disassociate myself from the pain and suffering. I couldn't anymore. If I continued to put myself in that position, I knew I wouldn't be able to deal with it. With that knowledge came a turning point for me. So I lay very still and willed the miles to be eaten in the heat of the turboprops.

It was eleven o'clock the next day when we set down

in Anchorage. Like an automaton, I carried out the rest of my duties. Finally, I was able to go back to where Barry was waiting. The minute he saw me, he could tell that something had happened. But a lot more had happened than just that one incident on Shimea. A lot had changed in me. To this day, the memory of John Sloane follows me around, a specter waiting just out of consciousness to remind me of my frailties.

They crept behind me, hiding in the shadows, all the way back to the house Barry and I had bought just outside Sacramento. It was the end of August, and I was so glad to see the dry, dusty hillside that I had to fight the tears welling behind my burning eyes. At home, Topah moved about the corral. The blaze on his forehead was like a beacon to me, saying, "Come. Hold me. Put your face against my neck. We're old friends."

I needed Topah, and I buried myself in his care. Barry and I built a barn, fixed a fence, worked on our house. From August to January I had opportinities to fly, and I was supposed to fly, but I didn't. Time went on until I was at the point where I had to fly again if I was to keep current with my standing. If I didn't take a mission very soon, I wouldn't be eligible to fly Air Evac anymore.

Somewhat reluctantly, I accepted a January flight to Chicago. Chicago was where it had all begun thirty years earlier. I hoped I could handle that flight. I could pretend that I was going home. But my home was on a ranch in the hills of California now, and I wasn't ready to take on the care of another patient. I felt as if I was being pulled from all sides.

Then Air Evac cancelled the flight. Without it, I would no longer be a flight nurse. I stared across the grounds in the direction of the runway. Full circle. And now, what would I do?

I wedged my things and myself into a phone booth and called Barry to tell him the Chicago mission had been cancelled.

Uneasiness rested uncomfortably in my chest. "But I have to fly, BC." I said.

A gentle and very sure voice crossed the telephone lines, and with one word, Barry gave me the answer to my problems.

"Why?" he asked.

Yes. Why? That was an out for me, a legitimate one. Why did I have to do it? Why couldn't I stop, now that it wasn't what I wanted? Why risk a severe burnout, one that I knew could cause some irreversible damage? John Sloane was still a vivid memory, one I had trouble putting in the past. Why get involved in something that I knew I might not be able to deal with? Why chance another John Sloane?

I needed to make peace with myself and my nursing career. I believed so completely in the importance of the profession, but at that time I needed to be more on the outside than directly involved in patient care.

So I left Air Evac on a bit of a negative note, but secure in doing so because it was with the understanding that it was better to get out than to stay in and be caught up in something critical that I couldn't deal with.

I don't regret for a moment having been in Air Evac. It was one of the most enchanting times of my life. I climbed a mountain and found it fulfilling. I could, indeed, look back and be proud. It was, as Commander West had promised, a right that I had earned. Yet, the price was very high. I suppose it's best summed up by a conversation I had with a doctor once many, many years before I even knew of Air Evac's existence.

This particular doctor was very talented, but also very

difficult to work with. He considered nurses as nothing more than servants to be used and thrown away without a care. Eventually it led to a confrontation where I had to defend myself and my profession—something I seldom found a need to do.

"Why, Drew," he'd asked, "is it such a big damn deal to be a nurse?"

Why? I stared at him for a second. Why? What did I say that he wouldn't have already discovered if only he'd only taken the time to open his eyes. Because nurses continually strive to do the impossible . . . because for every minute a doctor spends with a patient a nurse will put in a hundred . . . because we knew that if we didn't work ourselves above and beyond to stave off our patients' suffering, no one would . . . because when a nurse has given all she has to give, she has to dig deep within herself to find more . . . because we continually are the thin thread between life and death. In the end, I did nothing more than give him the chart he'd lost and that I'd spent forty valuable minutes searching for.

"Because," I said, "it's a noble profession."

Epilogue

It's been two years since I left Air Evac. I really miss everybody there. All the people I went in with are out now. All of my friends and I are married. We all came in single, and except for Mila, we all married someone we found in our own backyards, not really paying attention.

I hear that Virginia is married again and still busy climbing the ladder of success on everyone else's back—sometimes, even on her own. But that's Virginia.

I still fly, but now my husband is always the pilot and it's for pleasure, not a job. Barry came into my life and changed the way I see the world. Topah is getting older, but still has the regal gait of a champion. Our ranch is literally festooned with animals—horses, chickens, cats, and, now and then, even a skunk. So I guess the fortune teller was right.

The rest is just something we have to look forward to.

ACHEVÉ D'IMPRIMER
SUR LES PRESSES DE
L'IMPRIMERIE CHIRAT
42540 ST-JUST-LA-PENDUE
EN AVRIL 1994
DÉPÔT LÉGAL 1994 N° 8575

IMPRIMÉ EN FRANCE

NOTES

NOTES